nerve, muscle, and synapse

bernard katz
University of London

mc graw-hill book company
*New York   St. Louis   San Francisco
Toronto   London   Sydney*

mcgraw-hill series in the new biology

consulting editor: **george wald**

speakman: **molecules**

katz: **nerve, muscle, and synapse**

nerve, muscle, and synapse

Library of Congress Catalog Card Number 66-14815

10 11 12 13-MUMU-7 5 4 3 2 1

ISBN 07-033383-1

To my friend and teacher, A. V. Hill

foreword

When I first asked Professor Katz to write a book in this series, it was with the thought that it be primarily for such students as I have been teaching, mainly college freshmen and sophomores taking an introductory course in biology. We were already making good use of Katz's articles in the *Scientific American*, which we had found particularly informative and clear. I had hoped that in a short book he might extend the presentation at this level, with latitude not only to say what the subject contains, but to *teach* it.

Professor Katz has produced here the elementary text we asked of him, but also much more. He goes far beyond the first essentials to develop the subject in depth. He has the gift of a graphic style and the apt phrase. What impresses me particularly is that each idea is pursued to the numerical level. Each theoretical development comes out in this form, in clearly stated problems worked through with the relevant numbers. But the treatment as a whole extends beyond this also, asking and answering the basic questions that few workers in electrophysiology probably have taken the trouble to pursue so far. All this is done with an easy mastery of the underlying physics and physical chemistry.

I think therefore that there will be much here to interest and instruct a wide variety of readers, beginning with those for whom we had first intended the book, yet going beyond to advanced students, and, I suspect, mature research workers in the field. All of us in research work tend to leave gaps in our training, consoling ourselves with the thought that some day we will take the time to work through certain basic arguments that we have never quite mastered. Perhaps the principal contribution of this book is to raise such problems and see them through, on the way exposing facets of the subject that would otherwise have escaped our attention.

George Wald

preface

The purpose of this book is to explain in simple language what is known about the transmission of messages in the living body. It is not claimed that our present knowledge of the nerve signal and of the process of intercellular communication has as yet entered the orbit of "molecular biology." Nevertheless it is true that the exploration of nerve and muscle cells has advanced in recent decades and reached a point at which some of the biological processes can be described in physicochemical terms. Moreover, many of the elementary events are known from direct and quantitative observations on single cells, a procedure which has simplified the analysis and greatly aided our understanding.

Bernard Katz

contents

1

elements of
neuromuscular organization

Neuromuscular systems were developed early in the animal king-
dom; in fact, they were developed by the lowest multicellular
organisms in which tissue differentiation occurred. Even a seden-
tary sea anemone possesses specialized cells that make possible
sensory reception, rapid internal communication, and responsive
reflex movement when the animal is catching food or is in defensive
withdrawal.

There are, in principle, two mechanisms by which messages may
be transmitted within a living organism. One method depends on
the release of a specific chemical agent as a result, say, of a local
stimulus at point A. After circulating in the body, the substance
reacts at a remote site B, where some cell happens to be endowed
with a specific "receptor" molecule for this messenger. Certain
kinds of such messenger substances, called *hormones*, play an important part in regulating the metabolic effort of the organism. In
small unicellular animals, the release and internal diffusion or
circulation of chemical messengers could well be of major importance in the working out of quick reactions to external stimuli.
But in a large multicellular animal, in which different tissues have
developed specialized functions, efficient communication over long
distances could not be achieved by chemical messengers alone.
They could not provide the required speed and accuracy in regulating a vast traffic of signals or cope with the task of distributing
instant specific instructions to millions of different cells.

To execute these tasks is, of course, the function of the nervous
system in its various forms—from the relatively simple nerve net
of coelenterates to the immensely complex computer system of the
mammalian brain.

The successful development of even the simplest nervous apparatus
involves mechanisms the physicochemical nature of which we have
not even begun to guess. What are the guiding forces that cause

the axons of developing or regenerating nerve cells to grow, to travel long distances to their specific terminal stations, and among millions of cells to make contact with only a selected few? This is one of the most challenging questions in biology, and its importance is not diminished by the fact that we can give no clearer answer to it now than our predecessors could a hundred years ago.

It is customary to divide the nervous systems of higher organisms into two main parts—the peripheral apparatus and the central apparatus. The peripheral nervous system contains the long connecting cables (nerve fibers, or axons), each of which is the process of a centrally located cell. The function of the peripheral nerves is to transmit signals, rapidly and without fail—*afferent* signals from the sensory receptor organs which provide the input to the central computer system, and *efferent* messages going back to executive organs such as muscles and glands. The central nervous system— the spinal cord and brain—is a much more intricate apparatus and serves to sort and compare input signals, to coordinate them, and to work out suitable reactions. The importance and delicacy of this control system may be appreciated simply from the elaborate nature of its mechanical mounting; it is suspended in a shock-absorbing fluid medium within the protective bony structures of the skull and spinal canal.

All this together does not make up a complete nervous system; there are, in addition, concentrations of nerve cells distributed in the body (autonomic ganglia), whose input and output connections are relatively independent of brain control and which serve to provide automatic regulation of our internal organs and of the circulation of the blood.

In the invertebrate phyla one finds an organization of the nervous system that is somewhat different from ours. There, the sensory nerve cell bodies are situated in the periphery, near the actual points of reception of the sensory messages, and the motor nerve cells are concentrated in central ganglia together with the higher— integrating and coordinating—nerve cells.

The messages, then, which are carried by our peripheral nerves fulfill two main functions: they provide an input from sense organs and an output to skeletal muscles and glands. But to achieve fine and accurate control of muscular movement, provision is made for continuous automatic "feedback" of information and for constant reassessment and adjustment of motor reactions even after they have started. For this purpose, internal sense organs are built into our muscles and act as microscopic strain gauges, sending nerve messages to the centers by which the length and rate of movement of our muscle fibers are constantly monitored. The information derived from these *muscle spindles* is used to keep a constant check on the motor nerves and regulate automatically the stream of centrifugal impulses passing back to the muscles.

As a further refinement, the muscle spindles have built into them a sensitivity control consisting of fine specialized muscle fibers which are used to preset the tension on the sensory nerve endings. These fibers are under orders from the central nervous system, and depending on whether the muscle strain gauges are stiffened or slackened, this whole intricate system of reflex control can be alerted or "stood at ease." This is only one example of the many exceedingly subtle biological interactions, or servomechanisms, in which peripheral sense organs and central nerve cells are linked in order to achieve smooth, accurate, and automatic performance. As everyone knows, the proper use and the accurate timing of this apparatus have to be learned. Smoothness and accuracy of muscular movement are acquired only by practice. The mechanics of this process of learning how to time nerve impulses and how to make a highly complex motor action effortless and automatic are unknown; this is another of the fascinating and so far quite unsolved problems of neurophysiology.

The structural unit of our communication system is the individual nerve cell, or neuron, which contains a nucleus and cell body from which has grown a tree of many branches and twigs spreading in various directions (Fig. 1). Each nerve cell, in a way, is a nervous system in miniature: it receives afferent messages from many other neurons through their fine terminal contacts, or *synapses*, which are found on the cell body and its nearby dendritic processes. It sifts and integrates these signals and prepares suitable output messages which are passed on, along an efferent channel known as the *axon*, to the next sorting station.*

* The word "axon" is used for two purposes. (1) It is synonymous with "peripheral nerve fiber," that is, the enormously elongated peripheral process of a nerve cell [connected to a sense organ (afferent) or to a muscle (efferent)]. (2) It denotes the efferent channel of central neurons, that is, the cell process in which output signals travel away from the cell body.

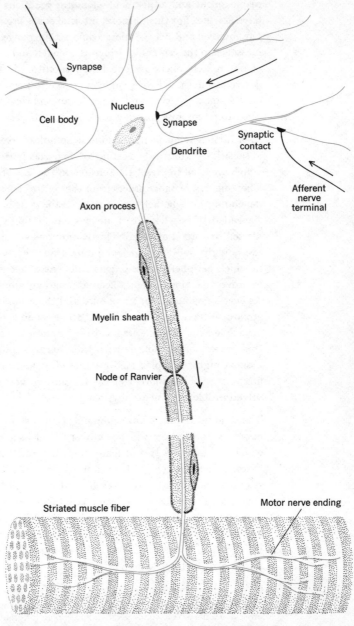

figure 1

Diagram of a nerve cell (spinal motor neuron of a frog) with some of its central (synaptic) and peripheral (neuromuscular) contacts.

To summarize the situation, we may state that *reception* of signals occurs at special contact points of the nerve cell body and its dendrites, *integration* of input signals takes place in the same region, within the surface membrane of the cell body, and the *response*, the initiation and onward travel of efferent messages, is the function of the axon.

The mechanism that enables nerve cells to perform these three important functions has been explored successfully, and a large part of the following chapters will be devoted to a detailed review of this recently acquired knowledge.

the structural relation between a nerve cell and its neighbors

It is not just at the synapses, where transmission of signals takes place, that nerve cells make intimate contact with other cells. The greater part of the neuronal surface is covered by closely apposed cells (known as satellite, glia, or Schwann cells), whose function is still a mystery.

The association between the nerve cell and its immediate neighbors is much closer than that between adjacent muscle fibers, which are separated by a small space containing collagen and other connective tissue fibrils. It is possible for experimental purposes to free single muscle fibers and work on them in isolation. In the case of nerve fibers, this is—strictly speaking—not feasible, and the many important experiments which have been made on single isolated axons have, in fact, been carried out on nerve cell processes which were surrounded by an inseparable envelope of Schwann cells closely clinging to the axon surface.

It is possible in tissue culture to obtain "naked" axons, but during normal embryonic development the nerve cell and its processes are invariably invested with a thin layer of satellite cells. Until recently, the structural relation between these cell components has been the subject of a perennial controversy.

The very concept of "individual" neurons—of neurons as separate and complete cell units—was challenged by an important school of histologists led by Hans Held, who insisted that the growing axon process actually invades the cytoplasm of the cells with which it associates and that in effect the whole nervous system forms a large syncytial* unit (neurencytium) and establishes cytoplasmic

* A "syncytium" is a mass of cells that are interconnected by fine cytoplasmic processes.

continuity with the tissues whose activity it controls. Opposed to this was the view of Ramón y Cajal, who maintained that nerve cells, although they form close contacts with other cells, are structurally separated from them and from one another and that the cytoplasmic contents of the contacting cells remain enclosed within isolating cell membranes. The historical controversy between the neuronal "contact" and neurencytial "continuity" theories was finally resolved in favor of Cajal's interpretation by the use of the electron microscope with its greatly increased resolving power.

It turned out that nerve cells and axons are almost completely enveloped by satellite (glia and Schwann) cells but that each cell is separate from its neighbor and there is a small gap between adjacent membranes, usually one hundred to a few hundred angstrom units wide.* Viewed in cross section, the Schwann-cell envelope of a peripheral axon process is generally so close and complete that it is easy to understand Held's firm belief that the growing axon penetrates the interior of the Schwann cells, and it is perhaps natural that there should have been a long and bitter dispute between the two rival theories, which were based (as many theories are) on the interpretation of structures just beyond the resolving power of the scientific instruments then available.

There has been much speculation concerning the function of these satellite cells and their possible participation in the process of nerve signaling. The question is sometimes posed whether the nerve impulse itself may not be produced by the Schwann-cell layer rather than by the axon. This is most unlikely. A great deal is known about the physical and chemical basis of the action potential and the propagation of this electrical wave along nerve and muscle fibers, and it is clear that the mechanisms in both cases are substantially identical and reside in the cylindrical fiber membrane. Muscle fibers lack Schwann cells and are invested very sparsely, at most at a few scattered places, with satellite cells of any description. The greater part of the muscle surface membrane is not associated with that of other cells, and yet the muscle fiber is capable of producing the same kind of self-propagating electric signal as that of a nerve axon. In certain invertebrate ganglia, it has been possible to place separate recording electrodes into the nerve cells and into the surrounding glia cells (Kuffler and Potter,

---

* The angstrom unit (Å) is 10^{-8} cm.

1964). In these cases, it could be shown directly that impulses are generated only within the neuron itself and not in the satellite cells.

A second suggestion that has been advanced is that the glia cells which surround the central nerve cell bodies may be concerned not so much with initiating or transmitting rapid signals, but with long-term storage of information, that is, with "memory" at the cellular level. This idea is not altogether unattractive, but at present the only feature which can really be said to be shared by memory and glia is that very little is known about either of them.

When a nerve is cut and its axons are thereby severed from their parent cell bodies, the peripheral axon processes cease to conduct impulses after a few days. Their structure disintegrates, and the remnants appear to be digested by the surrounding Schwann cells, which multiply and take up the spaces formerly occupied by the axons. At the same time, the central stump of each truncated nerve fiber tends to grow toward the periphery at a rate of a few millimeters per day and after resuming contact with the peripheral satellite cells, gradually begins to restore the original channel of communication with muscle fibers or sensory cells. The process of regeneration is controlled principally by the activity of the nucleus of the cell, and, what is more, the normal maintenance of the whole long peripheral axon depends on the integrity of the cytoplasmic connection with the cell body and its nucleus.

It has been suggested that the nucleated Schwann cells which surround the axon all along its length subsidize the axon metabolically and somehow make up for the fact that the nerve cell process is so far away from its own nucleus. (In terms of transport by ordinary thermal diffusion the peripheral axon terminals in long neurons are months or years away from the center.) This is a plausible suggestion; it makes it easy to see why similarly elongated muscle fibers which have an ample built-in supply of nuclei distributed along their cytoplasm can do without an investing sheath of nucleated satellite cells. It must, however, be remembered that Schwann cells are not capable by themselves of preserving the function and structural integrity of amputated axons, and, indeed, after a few days they start disposing of the axon remnants. The essential center for supply and maintenance of the axon is the nerve cell body and its nucleus, and it remains a challenging problem to find out how the neuronal nucleus manages to replenish

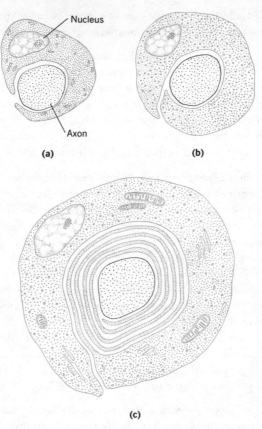

(a) **Cross section of nerve fiber (axon) and Schwann cell.**
(b) **and** (c) **show the development of the myelin sheath.**

the peripheral ends of the cell and keep them supplied with the required enzymes or with the tools for manufacturing enzymes on the spot. Presumably the essential substances are continually transported along the axoplasm and continually used up in the periphery. Whether the transport mechanism is related to the slow forward movement and longitudinal growth that one observes during regeneration of a severed stump or whether it depends upon a quite different and perhaps much faster physicochemical mode of propagation is not yet known.

In one special instance, the function of satellite cells is now well understood. Schwann cells are responsible for the formation of the myelin sheath, the insulating jacket found in all high-speed motor and sensory nerves of vertebrate animals. The work of Geren (1954), Schmitt (1959), and Robertson (1960) has shown that during embryonic and postnatal development, Schwann cells rotate around and around the nerve fiber, each ultimately forming a cylindrical bead consisting of many turns of its own cytoplasm and membrane wound tightly around the axon surface (Fig. 2) and covering one or a few millimeters of the axon length. The nerve membrane remains exposed only at the *nodes of Ranvier*, which are small gaps (each about 1 μ)* between adjacent segments of myelin.

The provision of this segmented sheath has been of the greatest importance in the development of the nervous system; it has—as we shall see—enabled animals to increase greatly the number of their fastest signaling channels without making extra demands on "cable space." The myelinated segments of our nerve fibers are the nearest biological approach to submarine cables (on a miniature scale), in which electric signals are conducted along the cylindrical axon core, which is separated from the conducting tissue fluid by a concentric insulating sheath. However, the most important structural component of a nerve fiber is not its myelin sheath, but the axon membrane which is exposed at the nodes of Ranvier. This is the site of *electric excitation*, an essential biological process by which automatic reinforcement of the nerve signal is brought about.

For well over a century, it has been known that the activity of nerves and muscles is intimately associated with the production of electric currents. We know now that the electric signal (action potential, or spike) which the physiologist has been recording from active nerve axons and muscle fibers is not just a by-product, but is the essential feature of the self-propagating message, the nerve *impulse*.

* 1 micron (μ) = 10^{-4} cm.

2
electricity and
neurophysiology

The development of our present-day concepts of nerve activity has depended very largely on improvements in electrical and electronic techniques. If one goes back to the eighteenth century, one finds that even in the early days of the history of electricity our knowledge of it was closely interwoven with studies of nerve and muscle. Long before the announcement of Ohm's and Faraday's laws, before the invention of galvanometers and other sensitive recording instruments, Luigi Galvani had discovered a form of electric discharge which he believed to be due to the production of electric currents by living nerve and muscle tissue. His interpretation was soon challenged by Alessandro Volta, who showed that the electromotive force in most of Galvani's experiments originated at the contact points between tissues and metals. The famous dispute between Galvani and Volta proved to be the impetus for a whole stream of experiments and ideas—in physiology as well as physics and physical chemistry— which have continued to grow and develop ever since.

For many years, the twitch that one observes when a brief current is discharged through the isolated nerve-muscle preparation of a frog was the most sensitive detector for short-lasting electric pulses. By the middle of the nineteenth century, Matteucci and Du Bois Reymond had discovered with the help of slow but sensitive galvanometers that nerves and muscles are capable of generating electromotive forces themselves. Thus, if one crushes one part of a nerve or muscle, the injured region becomes electronegative with respect to the undamaged parts and electric current will flow from the tissue through a galvanometer connected to it. Du Bois Reymond also showed that when a muscle responds to a series of electric shocks applied to its nerve, this is accompanied by a transient electric change in the muscle tissue which always consists of a reduction of the "injury current." The methods of recording then available were far too slow to reveal the true time course of the brief electric impulses which are associated with the activity of nerve and muscle fibers. By various ingenious procedures, Du Bois Reymond and, later, L. Hermann and J. Bernstein were able to find out that the electric activity of the cells occurs in the form of brief electric discharges, each of them lasting only a few thousandths of a second. But the physiologists had to wait for the invention of the cathode-ray tube (Fig. 3) and the thermionic amplifier to obtain accurate and direct measurements. The cathode-ray tube is an instrument capable of following instantaneous potential changes (more rapid than one is likely to encounter in living cells), but it is very insensitive, and one needs many volts to deflect the fast-moving electron beam sufficiently. Hence, the small signal (often much less than 1/1000 volt) that one wants to pick up from the tissue must be passed through several stages of amplification before it is large enough to be registered as a sizable deflection on the screen of the cathode-ray tube.

some technical matters It sometimes happens that in making the connections between the tissue and the amplifier and oscilloscope, the experimenter unwittingly introduces artificial time lags which distort and slow down the signal and so loses many of the benefits which the recording instrument was meant to provide. This is quite an im-

figure 3

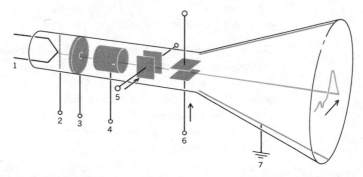

Cathode ray oscilloscope. The cathode (1) emits electrons. Control grid or "brightness control" (2) governs strength of electron current. Main anode, or "gun" (3), accelerates electrons. Focussing anode (4) forms sharp electron beam. Pair of horizontal deflection plates (5) produce "time base" deflection. Pair of vertical deflection plates (6) receive nerve signal from amplifier. Metallized screen (7) discharges electron beam after it has produced bright spot by collision with fluorescent screen on front of tube.

portant point, and to understand it we must go back to some elementary electric circuitry.

Suppose the signal generated by the tissue is a very rapid "square wave" of potential change, 1 msec in duration and 1 mv in amplitude, like the pulse shown in the diagram (Fig. 4a). In actual fact, living cells do not produce signals of such instantaneous rise and fall, but for the present purpose this is a simple case to discuss. Also, it is easy to generate signals of a similar kind artificially, for instance, by tapping a Morse key or by triggering a suitable electronic pulse generator. Suppose we want to display the signal on a cathode-ray tube whose deflection sensitivity is 0.5 mm/volt. If one were to apply the signal directly to the vertical pair of deflection plates, the spot on the screen would move by only 0.5 μ. To obtain a reasonable excursion of, say, 1 cm, the signal must be amplified 20,000 times; this can easily be achieved by interposing several stages of amplifying thermionic tubes between the primary electrodes and the cathode-ray tube.

We use the horizontal deflection plates of the cathode-ray tube to give us a "time base." By applying to these plates a voltage that increases at a constant rate, the spot is swept across the tube, from left to right, at constant speed. When the spot reaches the end of the traverse, the voltage is very rapidly switched off and the spot "flies back" to the left. It is possible to synchronize sweep and signal so that the latter appears at a suitable selected moment of the horizontal traverse and is displayed as a simple wave in or near the center of the screen. In practice, this is usually done by stimulating the tissue (nerve or muscle) with an electric shock at an adjustable interval after the start of the sweep. If we drive the spot across the face of the tube repeatedly, say 20 times per second, and elicit the signal each time at the same moment during the traverse of the beam, we obtain a standing wave. Ideally, this wave should have precisely the same "square" shape as the original signal; in other words, the instantaneous rise and fall of the pulse should be recorded faithfully without distortion. In practice, this is not always easy to achieve. Suppose that the tissue which generates the signal has a very high internal resistance or that one of the connecting electrodes has a high resistance, for example, 20 megohms. Suppose further that the input tube of the amplifier, or the leads connecting it to the tissue, has an appreciable inter-

figure 4

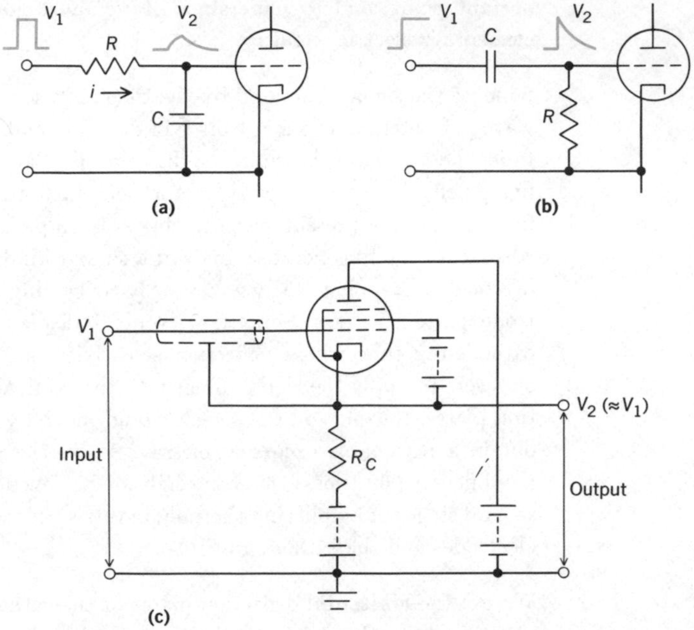

(a)

(b)

(c)

Diagrams at top show two kinds of signal distortion $(V_1 \to V_2)$. (a) This type can be caused by excessive resistance R in the nerve or in the recording electrode coupled with stray capacitance C between grid and cathode. (b) This type can arise from a polarization capacity of the electrode C coupled with a leak resistance R between grid and cathode. (c) The "cathode-follower stage," which reduces the effect of leakage (capacitative or resistive) between input grid and cathode. An input signal ΔV_1 alters the current flow Δi through the tube. This in turn produces an output signal $(\Delta V_2 = iR_c)$ which practically "follows" ΔV_1 and so automatically backs off the voltage change (and any accompanying current flow) between grid and cathode.

The following relations obtain where V_g is the potential difference between grid and cathode.

$$\Delta V_1 - \Delta V_2 = \Delta V_g$$

Also

$$\Delta V_2 = \mu \frac{\Delta V_g \, R_c}{R_c + R_a}$$

where μ is the voltage amplification factor and R_a is the internal resistance of the tube. Then

$$\Delta V_2 = \mu \frac{(\Delta V_1 - \Delta V_2) \, R_c}{R_c + R_a}$$

Suppose that the cathode load resistance R_c is made equal to R_a and μ is 50. Then

$$\Delta V_2 = 25 \, (\Delta V_1 - \Delta V_2)$$

$$\frac{\Delta V_2}{\Delta V_1} = 0.96$$

That is, the cathode voltage "follows" the grid voltage with 96% accuracy.

electrode capacity, say, 100 pf [1 pf (picofarad) = 1 $\mu\mu$f (micro-microfarad) = 10^{-12} f]. This means simply that the insulating material between the input electrodes (air or solid insulator between wires and vacuum between grid, cathode, and anode of input tube) behaves like the dielectric between the plates of a condenser and tends to absorb electric charge and allow a transient displacement current to flow when a quick potential change occurs between the electrodes. If this happens, the sharp edges at the beginning and end of the voltage signal will fail to appear on the cathode-ray tube. They will be rounded off as shown in the diagram, because, in effect, the input capacity acts as a momentary shunt through which current flows at the beginning and end, and only when this condenser has been fully charged up, or discharged again, will the full potential change be recorded. This process takes time;* it follows an exponential course with a *time constant* given by the product of the tissue-plus-electrode resistance and the input "shunt capacity." The product of 1 ohm × 1 f, or 1 megohm × 1 μf, is 1 sec. Hence, in our example, 20 megohms × 100 pf = 2 msec; this means that our signal would be badly distorted and attenuated.

There are several ways of avoiding this type of distortion. First one must recognize its existence. To do this, it is necessary simply to calibrate the recording system properly by applying a voltage pulse of known wave form and amplitude in place of the input signal and comparing it with the size and shape of the wave recorded on the cathode-ray tube. To overcome the distorting effect of the

* If a voltage "step" of amplitude V_1, in volts, is applied as in Fig. 4a, the voltage V_2 appearing between grid and cathode is given by

$V_2 = V_1 - iR$

where i = current, amp
 R = resistance, ohms

Also

$$i = C \frac{dV_2}{dt}$$

where C = capacity, f
 t = time, sec

Hence

$$V_2 = V_1 - RC \frac{dV_2}{dt}$$

the solution being

$$V_2 = V_1 \left[1 - \exp\left(-\frac{t}{RC} \right) \right]$$

input capacity, one uses short connections and a special input stage called a *cathode follower* (Fig. 4). For this purpose, a thermionic tube is used with the "load resistance" placed between cathode and high tension supply. The grid lead is usually surrounded by a shield which is also connected to the cathode. This arrangement causes the voltage signal to be passed on to the next stage without amplification, but also without serious distortion. This result is obtained because each time a voltage signal occurs at the grid electrode of the tube, the potential at the cathode changes "in step" by nearly the same amount;* the cathode potential *follows* the grid potential. As a consequence, practically no current can flow across the input capacity (as the voltage across it does not change appreciably), and the deleterious effect of the capacity is thereby neutralized. The output resistance of the cathode-follower stage is very low, and one can therefore use quite long leads to connect it to the next stage without distorting the signal. (Remember it is the product of resistance and capacity which matters.) There are a number of more elaborate methods of automatically compensating for input distortion; only a very elementary description has been given here.

In the context of a discussion of technical matters, it may be of interest to say a little more about amplifiers, stimulators, and electrodes.

If one wanted only to record the brief electric signals produced by nerve and muscle cells, it would be sufficient and convenient to use a capacity-coupled amplifier in which the high-tension supply of each stage is insulated from the input of the next stage by means of condensers which are interposed between the anode of one amplifying tube and the grid of the next one. Such condenser coupling simplifies the design of the amplifier and of its voltage supply, but it restricts the experimenter's choice and does not enable him to record slow potential changes or steady potential differences (p.d.'s) between different regions of cells or tissues. The reason, of course, is that the coupling condensers not only block the undesirable transfer of steady high voltages, supplied by the power pack, from one tube to the next, but they also prevent the transfer

---

* For example, if V_1 (Fig. 4c) becomes more positive, the current through the tube increases, causing V_2 also to become more positive. The larger the amplification factor of the tube, the more closely will the changes of V_2 follow those of V_1.

of steady or slowly changing biological p.d.'s from one stage of the amplifier to the next. To record such slow or steady electric phenomena, one must use a direct-coupled (or D.C.) amplifier in which the operating voltages supplied to the different stages must be carefully designed and balanced, since they all affect one another. A suitably constructed direct-coupled amplifier enables one to record faithfully all potential changes that one is likely to encounter in nerve and muscle cells; it covers a sinusoidal frequency range from "zero" (i.e., a steady p.d.) up to about 20,000 cycles per second.

It is necessary once again to use the right input connections and calibrate them, for otherwise the benefits of a good direct-coupled amplifier might easily be wasted. If one wants to record steady p.d.'s, it is important to use so-called *nonpolarizable* electrodes (e.g. chloridized silver wires dipped in a chloride solution). It is also important to select an input tube which has an almost infinite resistance between grid and cathode; this enables one to amplify and record p.d.'s without drawing any electric current from the tissue.

If one uses blank, polarizable metal electrodes and an input tube which has a slight leak between grid and cathode, the consequence is that any p.d. in the tissue causes current to flow through the recording electrodes and the leak resistance. This causes polarization at the junction between metal electrodes and tissue fluid, and within a short time these polarizable junctions will be charged up and produce an opposing electromotive force (emf) which blocks the continued transfer of steady or slowly changing tissue potentials. Polarization is, in fact, equivalent to a form of capacity coupling at the metal/electrolyte junction, and the advantage of the specially designed direct-coupled amplifier may therefore be lost. The "capacity effect" arises from the discontinuity between two types of carriers of electric current: electrons in the metal and ions in the electrolyte solution. The junction acts like an insulating barrier where electric charges accumulate and gradually build up a counter emf.

It should be noted that this kind of capacitative distortion and blockage of slow signals is the opposite of the capacitative shunting of fast signals which we previously considered. The difference is best visualized with the help of the diagrams in Figs. 4a and 4b.

In the previous case (a), an invisible stray capacity was *shunting* the input leads and caused rapid potential changes to bypass the amplifier. In the present case (b), another invisible capacity (due to electrode polarization) makes itself felt, but this time *in series* with the amplifier input; it allows rapid signals to get through, but opposes the transfer of slow potential changes or steady p.d.'s. The effect depends on the rate at which the surface capacity of the metal electrodes is charged up, in other words, on the amount of current flowing through the electrodes. This is controlled by the leakage resistance between grid and cathode of the input tube; the product of R and C determines the time course of the charging process and consequently the time when the transfer of a persistent voltage change is effectively cut off. Suppose $C = 1$ μf and R is very high (say 10,000 megohms); then no appreciable polarization will occur, and quite slow potential changes lasting many seconds may be recorded with ordinary wire electrodes. But if the leak resistance has a value of 1 megohm, the time constant RC is reduced to 1 sec and long-lasting potential changes will no longer be recorded. There are other reasons that make it troublesome to use blank wire electrodes for the recording of slow or steady potentials; the junction between metal and fluid is itself the site of a p.d. that tends to be rather unstable and fluctuates during, for example, local variations of oxygen pressure.

For these reasons it is preferable to employ reversible or non-polarizable electrodes (for example, calomel half-cells or chloridized silver wires), in which electric current can be carried continuously across the metal/electrolyte junction by means of a reversible chemical reaction.

In the case of a silver/silver chloride electrode the reaction can be written as

$$Ag + Cl^- \rightleftharpoons AgCl + \text{electron } \epsilon^-$$

or alternatively,

$$AgCl \rightleftharpoons Ag^+ + Cl^-$$
$$+\epsilon^- \Updownarrow -\epsilon^-$$
$$Ag$$

A coat of AgCl, whose solubility is very low, is deposited on the silver metal. It provides a solid store of Ag^+ and Cl^- ions and mediates between electronic conduction in the metal ($Ag^+ + \epsilon^- \rightleftharpoons$ Ag) and ionic current (owing to Cl^- exchanging between precipitate and solution). A system of this kind is often called a *chloride electrode*, or an electrode *reversible to chloride ions*. The important net result of the electrode reaction is that two-way flux of electric charge can take place—from electrons in the metal to chloride ions in the solution and vice versa. Consequently the flow of charge is relatively unimpeded by polarization, and current can be passed without building up a large counter emf (within limits set by the surface area of the electrode and by the concentration and mobility of the ions).

Electrodes of this type are not completely free from deficiencies and polarization effects. They have an appreciable resistance and generally can carry only small currents. During prolonged current flow, the chloride concentration around the metal/liquid junction slowly changes, and this is accompanied by a gradual rise of a small counter emf. (The electrode potential varies, as will be seen later, with the logarithm of the Cl^- concentration.) This effect, however, is usually quite small, and provided the coating of AgCl has not been allowed to disintegrate, the silver chloride electrode may be regarded as effectively nonpolarizable.

electric stimulation   In physiological experiments, electrodes are used for two principal purposes—for recording bioelectric signals and potential differences and for the stimulation of nerve and muscle cells.

The fact that nerve and muscle fibers are far more sensitive to electric currents and more easily excited by electric shocks than by other forms of stimuli is of great interest and was, of course, recognized by such early pioneers in the field as Galvani. The significance of the two outstanding properties of nerve, namely, excitability by electric currents and production of electric currents by excitation, was fully appreciated by the nineteenth century physiologists. L. Hermann pointed out that the current produced by an excited nerve would probably be sufficient to restimulate adjacent parts of the fiber and cause the excitation to propagate from point to point.

A great deal of work has been done in studying the detailed laws of electric stimulation to find out what kind of electric current pulses are most effective in eliciting a response and what the characteristic differences are in the electric excitability of different kinds of nerve and muscle fibers. It will be shown later that an electric stimulus produces its effect by rapidly discharging the surface membrane of the cell and reducing its existing p.d. to a lower unstable level at which excitation occurs. The current strength which is just needed to produce this effect is called the *threshold of excitation*. The cell membrane itself behaves like a leaky condenser with a time constant determined by its own resistance and capacity. A minimum quantity of electricity (that is, current intensity multiplied by time) must pass through it to change its potential with a brief current pulse. As one shortens the duration of a pulse, one must increase the current strength to maintain the efficacy of the stimulus. Such relations, when plotted graphically, are known as *strength-duration curves* (Fig. 5). With square pulses of long duration, a minimum current strength is needed below which excitation cannot occur. This is because the membrane capacity is leaky, and an absolute minimum of current strength is required to produce the necessary displacement of the membrane potential across the leak resistance.

figure 5

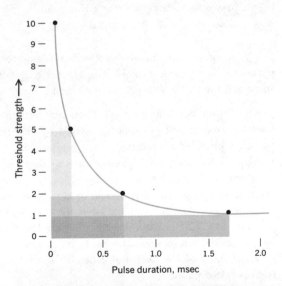

Strength-duration curve, showing the relation between the duration of a stimulating current (square wave) and the current strength needed to produce a nerve impulse. The "intensity × time" areas of 3 of the square-wave stimuli are also indicated.

A further property of all excitable cells is that they "accommodate" or "adapt" sooner or later to the change produced by an applied stimulus. In the case of electric excitation, this means that a constant current is effective when it is applied initially but loses its effect during its continued passage. A current of slowly rising strength may be imperceptible and not set up an impulse, even though it may rise gradually to an intensity many times greater than that at which a quickly rising square pulse is effective.

For the same reason, sinusoidal alternating current of very low frequency is ineffective because the rate of change of the current intensity is too low. An alternating current of very high frequency is also ineffective because its half-cycles are too brief to displace the membrane potential (the small effect of each half-cycle tends to be canceled by the next half cycle during which current flows in the opposite direction). In other words, at very high frequencies the membrane voltage cannot follow the applied current and the displacement of membrane potential is small. It is a curious fact that the most effective, and therefore also the most dangerous, form of electric stimulation is provided by the domestic and industrial alternating current supply, that is, sinusoidal waves at a frequency of 50 to 60 cycles per second.

In subsequent chapters, electric stimuli are frequently referred to without detailed description. These are usually brief shocks or square pulses lasting less than 1 msec, which are produced by electronic trigger circuits in which radio tubes or transistors are used to switch a current quickly on and off at desired time intervals. The current pulse is fed into the nerve through two electrodes which can again be of the polarizable (i.e., blank metal) or nonpolarizable (i.e., metal coated by one of its salts which can reversibly exchange ions with the solution) type. If one wants to apply a prolonged current of constant strength, it is best to use the reversible (nonpolarizable) kind of electrode and to place a high resistance in series so that any small changes of electrode resistance due to residual polarization effects cannot affect the current intensity appreciably. For many purposes, however, blank platinum wires can be used and are, in fact, preferred when one simply wants to apply brief stimulating pulses whose exact shape does not matter and which remain effective even if they suffer considerable distortion at the metal/liquid junction.

some electro-
physiological
observations

To introduce the subject to those who are not familiar with the basic language of the physiologist, it may be useful to describe some simple electrophysiological experiments. To begin with, we will use the simple method of working on a whole nerve containing many fibers in parallel, such as the isolated sciatic of a frog. Later, we shall describe experiments on single fibers. These are technically more difficult but have the great advantage that their results are easier to understand and much simpler to interpret!

If one dissects a frog nerve and places it in Ringer's solution (containing mainly 0.7% NaCl plus a little CaCl₂ and KCl), the nerve will survive in this medium for many hours or even days; that is, it remains capable of producing propagated electric signals which cause twitching in any attached muscle fibers and, of course, can be recorded with our amplifier and oscilloscope. We lift the nerve out of the solution and place it on two pairs of electrodes inside an airtight moist chamber, in which the nerve will retain a surface film of Ringer's solution without drying up. One pair of electrodes is connected to a pulse stimulator; the other, to our recording instrument.

We start by applying a series of very weak shocks—too weak to excite the nerve fibers. The arrangement one usually chooses is to drive the cathode beam across the tube at the same frequency (say 5/sec) at which the shocks are applied. By electrically controlling the time interval between the beginning of the horizontal sweep voltage and the shock, one can display the latter as a small vertical deflection during the early part of the horizontal traverse, always in the same position on the screen. This deflection is called the "stimulus artifact": it is simply a small leakage from the pulsing unit that is picked up by the amplifier just as electric interference from various kinds of pulse or spark generators is picked up by a television broadcast receiver. The stimulus artifact, provided it is not too large, is very useful, since it serves as a marker of the precise time at which the pulse was sent through the nerve. If one gradually increases the intensity of the stimulus, the size of the artifact also increases, and at a certain threshold strength a new kind of electric signal becomes noticeable that consists of a delayed small deflection (Fig. 6). This is the *response* of the nerve—the impulse or action potential—which is initiated at one of the stimulating electrodes and then travels at finite speed

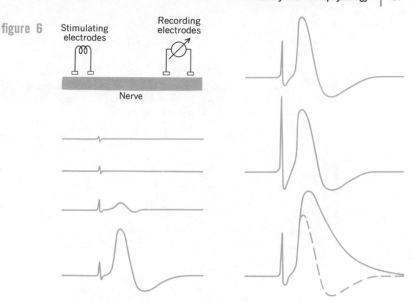

figure 6

Stimulating electrodes

Recording electrodes

Nerve

Action potentials recorded from an isolated whole nerve. The strength of the electric stimulus is increased in successive records starting at top left. The first two stimuli are below threshold strength. In the last record (bottom right), the "diphasic" action-potential wave has been changed to a "monophasic" wave. (This is done by placing the distal recording electrode farther away, at the dead end of the nerve.) See also Fig. 7.

toward the recording electrodes. The delay is due to the time taken up by the impulse in traveling from the point of initiation to the nearest recording lead. The signal consists of a wave of surface negativity lasting one or a few milliseconds; i.e., as the impulse passes a particular point of the nerve, the surface at that point becomes electronegative for a brief time with respect to regions further along (and not yet invaded). So at first the nearest electrode becomes negative relative to the more distant electrode; later the wave passes on to the distant electrode and this point becomes negative while the potential change at the first point is declining. The recorded result is a *diphasic* action potential (Figs. 6 and 7). If one prevents the impulse from reaching the second electrode, e.g., by damaging the nerve in the intermediate region or applying a paralyzing drug, only a simple *monophasic* wave of negativity may be recorded as the impulse reaches the first electrode and then dies out a little beyond.

Having reached the threshold point, we now increase our stimulus strength further and find that the amplitude of the action potential

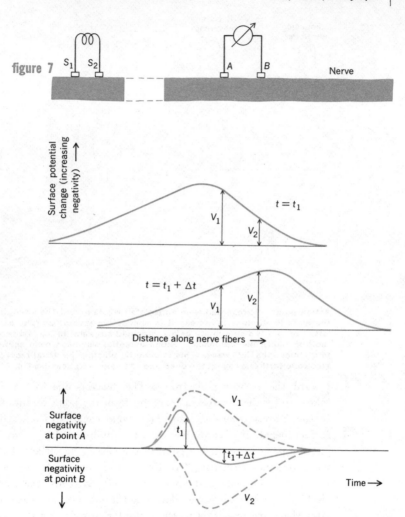

"Diphasic" action potential arises from superposition of waves of surface negativity, passing in succession the two points (A and B) at which the recording electrodes have been placed.

rapidly increases up to a maximum size beyond which further strengthening of the stimulus has no appreciable effect. The maximum amplitude may amount to some 15 or 20 mv; this figure varies greatly with the conditions of recording, for instance, with the thickness and length of the stretch of nerve between the electrodes.

Each time an impulse has passed, it leaves the nerve in a "refractory" state for one or a few milliseconds. During the first 1 or 2 msec the nerve is unable to conduct another signal, and it takes several milliseconds to recover the power of producing signals of full strength. If we apply, during each traverse of the cathode beam, a second shock at variable intervals after the first, we can determine the degree of recovery by measuring the amplitude of the second response (Fig. 8). With very brief intervals between shocks (1 to 2 msec), only the first impulse appears; with longer

figure 8

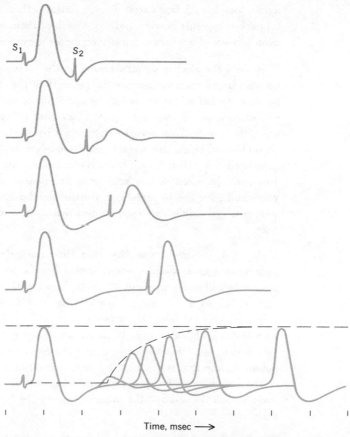

Time, msec ⟶

Refractory period as observed in an isolated whole nerve. In record at top, the second stimulus (S_2) is applied during the "absolute" refractory period, when it fails to excite any fibers. As the interval between S_1 and S_2 is increased, more and more fibers become excited a second time.

pauses, a second wave is observed that is small at first and then grows in amplitude as it is separated in time from its predecessor. This is a very important property of nerve cells: it means that their capacity of sending signals to distant points of the body is restricted to a series of brief standard pulses of limited frequency. The impulses may be compared to the standard elements of a signaling code (like the dots of the Morse system) in their usefulness to transmit information.

It is not easy to tell from a simple experiment of the type just described what the signals of the individual cells, i.e., of the single axons, look like. A frog's sciatic nerve contains thousands of fibers all packed together in one bundle, yet each of them represents the axon process of a separate sensory or motor nerve cell.

Why does the electric signal received at the recording electrodes become larger when we increase the strength of the stimulus? Is it because statistically more and more axons are being excited, each contributing an all-or-none bit (that is, a signal of fixed amplitude) when its threshold happens to be reached by the applied shock? Or do the individual fibers react more strongly and produce larger signals all along their length when the initiating stimulus is made stronger? Questions of this kind remained unanswered for many years and gave rise to prolonged, controversial arguments, which were resolved only when experimenters managed to work on single cells.

Today it is common knowledge that the propagated impulse in each axon is an all-or-none event arising from a potential change across the cell membrane, but 50 or 60 years ago this was far from certain. It is worth considering in a little more detail *why* the action potential recorded from the surface of a nerve bundle should vary with the stimulus intensity. What we are really recording in this case is not the potential change across the cell membrane but the potential drop that is produced by local currents along the outside of the active nerve fibers flowing from the resting regions in the front and in the wake of the impulse toward the forward moving active center.

The lines of current are shown in the diagram of Fig. 9. We are adhering throughout to the usual convention, namely, that the direction of electric current flow is from positive to negative potentials; i.e., currents flow along a falling gradient of potential. This happens to be the opposite of the direction in which electrons flow in a metallic conductor or in which negative ions flow in an electrolytic solution, and it coincides with the movement of positive ions (e.g., sodium and potassium) down a potential gradient. The convention regarding electric signs is very old; it antedates the discovery of ions and electrons, but as it is still generally used in textbooks of physics, it is also adopted here. Thus, when we speak for example of "inward" current flowing through the cell membrane, what we mean is simply an inward flow of positive charge or outward flow of negative charge. We do not imply anything about the species of ions carrying the current or about whether the current is due to ionic transfer through the membrane (ionic current), or to accumulation or depletion of ions on either side (capacity current).

During the passage of an impulse, action currents flow in local circuits (as shown in Fig. 9) from the active region along the inside of the axon, outward through the adjacent resting parts of the membrane, back along the external medium, and inward through the active membrane, so completing the circuit. As will be clear from the diagram, the *net* longitudinal current which flows through any one cross section is zero because at any point the currents

figure 9

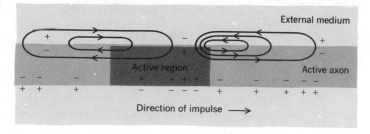

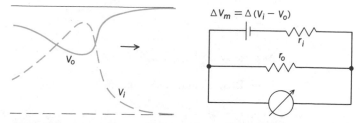

Recording with surface electrodes. The external potential change V_o is only a fraction of the total displacement of the membrane potential V_m. V_o arises from local currents flowing along the external medium (top diagram), causing a potential drop across the external resistance r_o (bottom diagram).

along the axon core are of equal strength and opposite direction to those flowing along the external fluid. But the *density* of the longitudinal current and the longitudinal p.d. between two points are not necessarily the same inside and out. The axial current inside is concentrated within the narrow tube of the axon cylinder, and the current along the outside is usually distributed among the interstitial fluid and among inactive nerve fibers. If only a few axons are active, the current produced by them will spread through the adjacent tissue and the external current density will be very low.

What we are really interested in is the potential change that takes place across the individual cell membrane (membrane potential $V_m = V_i - V_o$, where V_i is the potential on the inside and V_o that on the outside of the membrane). What we actually record from a whole nerve trunk is much less than this. By Ohm's law the current along the outside i_o is

1 $$i_o = \frac{-1}{r_o} \frac{dV_o}{dx}$$

where V_o = potential on the surface

$\dfrac{dV_o}{dx}$ = external potential gradient

r_o = resistance per unit length of the outside medium (including the shunt presented by inactive fibers)

The negative sign is in accordance with our convention and means that the direction of electric current is positive along a falling (negative) gradient of potential. The current along the inside i_i is, similarly,

2 $$i_i = \frac{-1}{r_i} \frac{dV_i}{dx}$$

As already explained, $i_o + i_i = 0$.

From Eqs. (1) and (2) we obtain

3 $$V_o = a - r_o \int i_o \, dx$$

and

4 $\quad V_i = b - r_i \int i_i \, dx = b + r_i \int i_o \, dx$

Here a and b are the constant levels of potential, outside and inside along the resting axon, with which we are not concerned at present. If we ignore these constants, Eqs. (3) and (4) give us the change of potential produced by the flow of longitudinal current along the axon core and along its outer surface.

The recorded potential V_o will start changing as soon as the impulse approaches the site of the nearest recording electrode and produces longitudinal current flow at this point.

From Eqs. (3) and (4) it follows that the change of membrane potential $V_i - V_o$ is

$$\Delta(V_i - V_o) = (r_o + r_i) \int i_o \, dx$$

while the recorded change of external potential V_o is

$$\Delta V_o = -r_o \int i_o \, dx$$

Hence, we observe only a fraction of the membrane potential change, namely

$$\frac{\Delta V_o}{\Delta(V_i - V_o)} = \frac{-r_o}{r_o + r_i}$$

Just as with an ordinary potential divider, we are monitoring a fraction that depends on the ratio between external shunt resistance r_o and the sum of the total—inside plus outside—resistances $(r_o + r_i)$.

Incidentally, the electric sign of the external potential change is negative-going, i.e., the opposite of the positive-going membrane potential change $V_i - V_o$.

If we record from the surface of a nerve bundle containing 1,000 identical fibers and the impulse in each fiber is accompanied by the same change $(V_i - V_o)$, the greater the number of synchronously excited fibers, the larger the externally recorded potential will become. The reason is that the ratio $r_o/(r_o + r_i)$ increases as more and more fibers actively contribute to the action current instead of being just passive external shunts.

Suppose each axon has associated with it a small amount of external shunting fluid whose resistance is equal to that of the axon core. Then, if all the 1,000 axons in our bundle produce a synchronous impulse, $r_o = r_i$ and the ratio $r_o/(r_o + r_i)$ will be 0.5, so we record one-half of the membrane potential change. If only 100 fibers are active, then r_i becomes 10 times larger than before and r_o will be reduced by a factor of 1,000/1,900 (because the 900 inactive cores contribute to the external shunt). Hence $r_o/(r_o + r_i)$ is now $(1/1.9)/(1/1.9 + 10) = 0.05$, instead of 0.5. Thus, one would expect the recorded potential to be proportional to the number of active fibers and, therefore, to vary with the stimulus strength, even though the response of each individual fiber may be a constant all-or-none phenomenon.

This conclusion, however, does not prove the all-or-none nature of the impulse. To obtain clear information on this point and to make more accurate measurements of the cellular membrane potential changes, a more direct approach involving the use of single cells must be chosen.

3

some observations on single nerve and muscle fibers

An isolated nerve or muscle, for instance the sartorius muscle of a frog or a giant nerve fiber from a squid, is placed in a suitable salt solution (a Ringer's solution containing 115 mM NaCl, 2 mM KCl, and 1.8 mM CaCl$_2$ for the frog muscle and ordinary sea water for the nerve fiber of a marine invertebrate like the squid). As before, we use two pairs of electrodes—one for stimulation and the other for recording purposes. The electrodes are chloridized silver wires that are connected (through agar-salt bridges) to different pipettes. One pipette of each pair consists of a very fine capillary whose tip diameter is small enough to allow one to insert it into the inside of a fiber. The other pipette is a tube of ordinary size that makes a fluid contact with the bath solution. One pair of electrodes is connected to a pulse stimulator which is used to deliver a stimulating current to the cell. The other pair is led from the cell to a cathode follower, voltage amplifier, and oscilloscope to register potential differences. The fine capillary pipettes have a tip size of about 0.5 μ or less. They are filled with a concentrated KCl solution which has two important advantages. First, the concentrated salt solution serves to keep the electrode resistance of the very fine micropipette as low as possible, although it can rarely be reduced much below 10 to 20 megohms. As has been pointed out previously (Fig. 4), a high electrode resistance can lead to serious distortion of the recorded signal, especially if the input tube of the amplifier presents a capacitative shunt. With electrodes of 10 to 20 megohms resistance, it is essential to use a cathode-follower stage which neutralizes current flow between grid and cathode and so enables the signal to be passed on with a minimum of distortion or attenuation.

The second advantage of the concentrated KCl solution is that it obviates "liquid junction" potentials, which arise from unequal mobilities of different ions at the boundaries of different electrolytes.

When two solutions containing different salts or unequal concentrations of the same salt come into contact, the solutes diffuse across the liquid boundary. Diffusion is a random process of thermal agitation, like Brownian motion, in which the elementary particles—molecules or ions—tend to move independently. If the positive ion of a salt has the greater mobility, it will tend to move ahead, down its concentration gradient, faster than its negative ion partner, but no substantial separation can occur because of the large electrostatic force of attraction that develops as soon as the process of diffusion begins. There will thus be a temporary balance between thermal agitation, which tends to separate ions of unequal speed, and electromotive force (diffusion potential or liquid junction potential), which tends to keep together ions of opposite charge. Diffusion potentials are, in general, much smaller (and so less liable to vary with temperature changes, etc.) than the electrode potentials that develop at a metal/liquid boundary or at the boundary between a silver-chloride or calomel electrode and the solution. It is therefore always desirable to make fluid contact with the nerve or muscle by means of a pipette and to keep the metal contacts well out of the way and in a constant environment. Even so, the liquid-junction potential can give rise to serious errors when, in the course of the experiment, the tip of the recording pipette is moved from the external solution into the interior of the cell with its quite different ionic composition. Indeed, this presents quite a serious problem and has given rise to a great deal of controversy regarding the interpretation of cellular potential measurements.

The use of concentrated KCl to overcome diffusion potentials is a well-established procedure and is based on the fact that potassium and chloride have nearly identical mobilities. Provided their concentrations are far above those of the solutes in the adjoining medium, the rate of diffusion of K^+ and Cl^- ions will swamp and short-circuit any p.d. that the other solutes would tend to produce. Difficulties can nevertheless arise with very fine micropipettes because the tips tend to clog with charged particles and then give erratic results. Careful selection of pipettes and frequent cross-checking of potential measurements with many different pipettes are therefore necessary.

After this technical digression, let us return to our experiment. We start with all electrodes in the salt bath. There will probably be a small p.d. between the two recording electrodes due to some asymmetry in the system, but provided the p.d. is steady, we may ignore it. We now move the fine recording probe up to a superficial fiber. At the moment of penetration one observes a sudden deflection on the oscilloscope. When the tip of the micropipette enters the cytoplasm, it finds itself at a lower electric potential—60 to 90 mv negative with respect to the outside bath. In general, this p.d. is maintained at a steady level so long as the microelectrode tip remains inside the fiber and provided that no stimulus is applied to the fiber or its neuronal connections. This is the "resting potential," which has been known to exist for more than 100 years, although it has previously been measured less accurately and through more indirect methods. The same p.d. is found at all points no matter where the electrode is inserted into the undisturbed resting cell. With certain interesting exceptions [e.g., at many synapses and motor end plates (Chap. 9)], potential differences have not been observed to occur *within* the cytoplasm, but only across the surface of the resting cell.

Continuing the experiment, we now employ the second pair of electrodes and pass a brief current pulse, say 10^{-7} amp strong and 2 msec long, with the fine pipette connected to the cathode of the pulse generator. The micropipette is moved toward the same fiber and eventually is made to penetrate the cell surface within a short distance, say 50 μ, from the previously inserted recording electrode. So long as the pulse pipette remains in the outside solution, no deflection is seen on the oscilloscope apart from a momentary "artifact" picked up through stray capacities at the beginning and end of the pulse. But when the pulse microelectrode enters, the current pulse passes across the high-resistant fiber surface and in doing so produces a large potential drop which is registered on the oscilloscope. This voltage signal has a characteristic rounded time course which differs from the instantaneous rise and fall of the applied "rectangular" current (Figs. 10 and 11). This subthreshold potential change, registered in the neighborhood of the stimulating electrode and not conducted, was known for a long time as the *electrotonic potential*, a somewhat archaic term, which is still being used for want of a better word.

The observations so far show us that the surface of the fiber contains a layer which is the site of a large potential gradient (the

figure 10

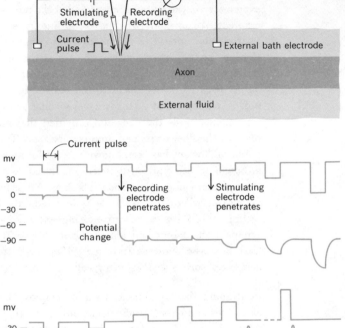

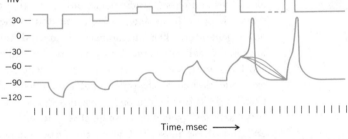

Time, msec ⟶

**Recording the membrane potential at the site of stimulation. The stimu-
lating and recording microelectrodes are inserted into the axon side-by-
side. Square current pulses are applied, producing "electrotonic" potentials and—if the current is strong enough and flows outward through the
axon membrane—giving rise to action potentials.**

inside being nearly 0.1 volt negative with respect to the outside)
and which has an electric resistance sufficiently high to give rise
to a large p.d. (of some 50 mv) when a small current (a few tenths
of a microampere) passes through it. If one alters the distance
along the fiber between the pulsing and recording micropipettes,
it is found that the voltage signal received by the latter rapidly
fades away, 50% attenuation occurring along every 1 to 2 mm.

Measurements of this kind have been used to determine the "cable constants" of the fiber and particularly the transverse leakage resistance of its surface membrane and the longitudinal resistance of the cytoplasm. The fact that the voltage signal has a slower rise and fall than the applied current pulse shows that the membrane

figure 11

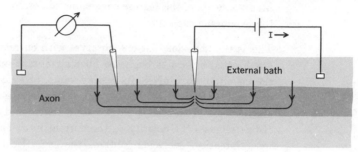

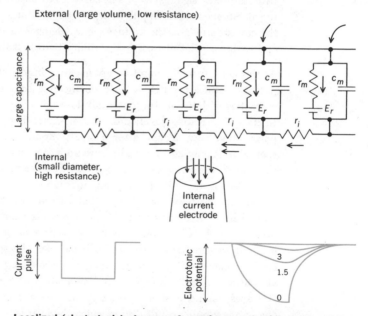

Localized (electrotonic) changes of membrane potential, produced by a current pulse. Diagram at top shows direction of current flow and the positions of current-passing and potential-recording microelectrodes, which are inserted close together in a single axon. The electric circuit (middle) represents distributed resistance and capacitance of axon core and axon membrane. Diagram at bottom shows square current pulse and resulting potential change across the membrane, recorded at 0, 1.5, and 3 "length constants" away from the current-passing electrode (see also page 73 and Fig. 18 below).

has a characteristic "charging-up" time. It has the property of a "leaky condenser," whose voltage lags behind the current passing through it with a time constant depending on the capacity as well as the resistance of the membrane. The further away one records the voltage signal from its point of origin, the slower it becomes. Measurements of this feature enable one to determine the value of the membrane capacity.

This is the behavior that one observes with current pulses which are directed inward through the fiber membrane and which raise the membrane p.d. above its resting value, or *hyperpolarize* it. If one doubles the strength of the pulse, the voltage signal also increases twofold and has a similar time course and spatial decay. If one reverses the polarity of the current pulse and uses a very weak intensity, one again obtains the same local phenomenon, with its electric sign reversed. The current flowing outward through the membrane reduces its p.d. or *depolarizes* it. But as one increases the current strength, the voltage signal changes in character and approaches a point of electric instability known as the *threshold*.

At this point (usually about 50 mv negative inside) the membrane potential passes through a state of unstable equilibrium. If the current is withdrawn, the potential does not immediately return to its stable resting level; one of two things happens. The depolarization may decline after a small variable delay (local response) or it may automatically flare up into a much larger potential change, the *action potential* or *spike*. This is a process no longer controlled by the initially applied current pulse; it is a transient self-amplifying potential change that exceeds the threshold displacement by a factor of 4 to 10 and crosses the zero line.* At its peak it reaches a level of 40 to 50 mv, *positive inside*, from which it rapidly swings back to the resting level. Once this spike potential has been elicited, it propagates along the whole length of the fiber at constant velocity and without attenuation of signal strength. It leaves behind a short refractory period—a silent interval of one or a few milliseconds during which the fiber is unable to carry a second signal. Thereafter the system is ready to be reexcited and to fire another propagated impulse.

* The "zero-line" is the steady *reference level* given by the potential of the solution on the outside of the fiber. When the internal potential reaches the zero line, the potentials inside and outside are equal.

If one records the electrical events at a sufficient distance (1 cm or more) from the point of stimulation, the subthreshold behavior is not seen at all. However, when the stimulus exceeds threshold, the propagating spike is received in full strength, its amplitude and shape being independent of the originating stimulus (Fig. 12). This phenomenon has been called "all-or-none response"; the term applies to the propagating spike of an individual cell recorded far away from its point of origin. It indicates that we are dealing with a triggered self-reinforcing event.

The procedures in the experiments just described could be queried on two grounds: (1) that an isolated tissue studied in an artificial environment may give abnormal reactions, and (2) that the introduction of micropipettes into a cell might seriously disturb the system which one wants to study.

It is quite true that isolated nerve and muscle tissues, even those of cold-blooded animals, are not in a perfect steady state. Over a

figure 12

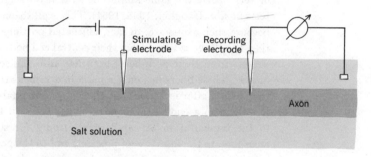

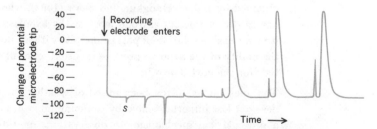

The response of a single axon. Stimulation and recording are done with the help of intracellular microelectrodes. The points of stimulation and recording are kept far apart. After insertion of the recording electrode, eight stimuli (very brief shocks, s) of varying polarity and intensities are applied. Provided the shock is of the right polarity and exceeds a critical threshold strength, an action potential of fixed magnitude (all-or-none response) results.

period of many hours they gradually deteriorate. (For example, they lose their potassium content and take up sodium from the surroundings; at the same time, resting and action potentials slowly diminish.) The rate of this running-down process depends on various factors, such as the experimenter's skill, adequacy of oxygen supply, thickness of tissue, and temperature and composition of the bathing solution.

Under suitable conditions, however, the tissue can be kept in a state sufficiently stationary for the requirements of our experiments. For example, isolated frog sartorius muscles can be maintained at low temperature (0 to 4°C) in Ringer's solution for some days, and give constant responses to electric stimulation (Hill, 1949), maintaining their potassium content at almost normal level (Ernst, 1958). Giant nerve axons of the squid can be isolated and kept in sea water at room temperature for several hours during which they are able to conduct several hundred thousand impulses of very nearly the same amplitude as that observed during initial tests *in situ* (Hodgkin, 1958, 1964). This is all the more remarkable because such axons are, in fact, mutilated portions of single cells; they have been severed from their central cell body and nucleus as well as from their peripheral branches and connections with the muscle. These fibers not only remain in a sufficiently normal functional state after isolation, but their large size enables one to subject them to a good deal of intracellular surgery, to cannulation, to the implantation of capillary electrodes for stimulation and recording, to the insertion of pipettes, and to the perfusion of their interior with artificial fluids. A dramatic result of this kind was obtained by Baker, Hodgkin, and Shaw (1962), who showed that one can mechanically extrude most of the axoplasm and replace it by a suitable solution of potassium salts without interfering with the ability of the axon to produce its usual series of action potentials for the next 3 or 4 hr.

The question has often been raised of whether the experimenter does not lose important clues by confining himself, in the study of a physiological mechanism, to observations on isolated tissues, cells, or cell fragments (such as an axon). There is no general answer to this question; by doing this, one is clearly removing important influences—e.g., the interactions between the axon and its cell nucleus or between the axon and its contacting nerve and effector cells, and of course any hormonal effects produced by remote tissues. Such influences are certainly of great importance for long-term processes of growth, repair, and replenishment of the cells we study. But it is equally clear that if one is concerned simply with the mechanism of the nerve signal and its transmission to and from muscle fibers, the maintenance of connections with other parts of the body is not required and in most cases would be an impossible impediment for the experimenter. The isolated axon has sometimes been likened to a system which has retained its storage battery, enabling it to draw current for many hours, but which is slowly running down in the absence of a recharging plant. Even this is not quite true, for the nerve fiber remains capable of "recharging its battery"; by using its enzymic metabolism, it can actively extrude sodium from the interior against electrical and concentration gradients (Hodgkin, 1958). So, if one looks for a crude analogy, it would be better to compare the isolated axon with a system that has kept both battery and trickle-charger; if it runs down slowly, this is for other reasons, perhaps partly because its fuel supply is not replenished and partly because of inadequate repair of its protein structure.

The second objection, namely, that intracellular pipettes have a disturbing influence, can be answered by relatively simple control experiments (in which, for example, the electrical behavior of the cell is monitored with one electrode during the insertion of a second electrode). In practice, penetration of the cell surface can be done satisfactorily if the tip of the pipette is very small, if the dimensions of the cell are large, and if the surrounding tissue does not interfere mechanically. Pipettes of 0.5-μ tip size, filled with a concentrated KCl solution, can be inserted into a 100-μ muscle fiber and kept there for many minutes without lowering the resting potential by more than 1 or 2% and frequently without leaving even a microscopic trace of local damage behind. But if one tries to use larger pipettes, one produces increasingly serious local damage as soon as the probe penetrates or scrapes against the cell membrane. The *advantages* of being able to record directly across the cell membrane are very great indeed. The development of the method of intracellular recording, together with the use of giant axons and tracer ions, was, in fact, the groundwork for the striking advances made in this field since 1939.

4

the membrane concept

The type of experiment just described shows that nerve and muscle cells are capable of storing electricity and of releasing electric energy in brief impulsive bursts. Living cells contain about 80% water with some electrolytes but no metallic conductors. It is clear therefore that we must look into the ionic makeup of cells and their surroundings before we can begin to understand the process by which electricity is generated in them.

Much of what follows will be drawn indiscriminately from experiments on nerve and muscle, especially on the large cephalopod axons (which are up to 1 mm thick in the squid) and on frog muscle. Nerve and muscle fibers, in spite of their different functions, have important features in common. They are both long cylindrical structures capable of propagating all-or-none impulses over the whole surface; by these means a momentary state of excitation is rapidly conveyed to the whole of the cell from end to end. In the nerve, this mechanism serves the purpose of transmitting signals rapidly between remote points; in skeletal muscle fibers the action potential acts as a stimulus, a precursor to contraction, and the fast propagation of the action potential ensures an almost synchronous development of tension all along the fiber. Nerve and muscle fibers share some other characteristic properties which are indicated schematically in Fig. 13. The distribution of electrolytes and the difference of electric potential between the cytoplasm and the surroundings are very similar in both cases.

In other respects there are important differences (some of them have already been mentioned). Thus a nerve fiber is a long cell process far distant from its nucleus but surrounded by a set of nucleated Schwann cells. The muscle fiber is a self-contained cell system with multiple nuclei distributed along its cytoplasm; its surface is generally "bare" or has only few scattered satellite cells attached to it (Katz, 1961). Its internal structure is much more highly organized—longitudinally into fibrils and orderly arrays of myofilaments and transversely into neatly aligned sarcomeres and their different crossbands.

The cytoplasm contains an aqueous protein gel, 10 to 20% of which is made up of solids, the rest being water. The water content of the cell can be altered by diluting or concentrating the outside salt solution. An isolated squid or cuttlefish axon adjusts its water content fairly rapidly and by swelling or shrinking reaches a new equilibrium within a few minutes. There has been much argument about whether the osmotic equilibration of the cell should be attributed to the presence of a semipermeable membrane or to the swelling and shrinking of the polyelectrolyte gel of which the cytoplasm is composed. Such swelling and shrinking would be independent of the presence of a surface membrane (see, for example, Katchalsky, 1954, or Ernst, 1958). Many investigators take the view (for example, Conway, 1950) that the structural proteins of the cell with their fixed electric charges and associated counterions make only a small contribution to the osmotic balance of nerve and muscle fibers, but the quantities are still uncertain.

Although the greater part of a nerve or muscle cell is taken up by water, which is in osmotic equilibrium with the surrounding tissue fluid, the chemical composition of the solutes, and in particular the electrolyte content of the cell, differs greatly from that of the external medium (Fig. 13). On the outside, the major ionic constituents are sodium and chloride; inside the cell, these ions amount to less than 15% of the electrolyte balance. Sodium is replaced by potassium, which is accumulated to a concentration approximately 20 to 50 times higher than in the external fluid. The intracellular anions have not been completely identified: in the giant axon of the squid, a special organic anion, isethionate, is present in a concentration of 270 mM; in other nerve fibers, glutamic and aspartic acids have been reported in substantial quantities. In muscle, Conway (1950) calculates that the negative charges are supplied largely by organic phosphates and amino acids and only about 10% are fixed to structural proteins, but Ernst (1958), Troschin (1958), and Ling (1962) maintain that the greater part of the internal negative charges are provided by the polyelectrolyte proteinates. Moreover, these latter authors take the view that the potassium ions do not merely form counterions to the negatively charged colloidal structure but possess selective affinity and are chemically bound to the proteinates.

figure 13

Frog muscle		Squid axon	
External	Internal	External	Internal
Na$^+$ 120	Na$^+$ 9.2	Na$^+$ 460	Na$^+$ 50
K$^+$ 2.5	K$^+$ 140	K$^+$ 10	K$^+$ 400
Cl$^-$ 120	Cl$^-$ (3–4)	Cl$^-$ 540	Cl$^-$ 40-100
	(A$^-$)		Isethionate$^-$ 270
			Aspartate$^-$ 75
	−90 mv		−60 mv

Electrolyte concentrations (mM/l) and potential differences across cell membrane.

It seems, however, very difficult to support this view in face of the following pertinent observations by Hodgkin and Keynes (1953). These results are discussed here in detail because they are of crucial importance in the still persistent argument about the validity of the membrane concept. Hodgkin and Keynes studied (a) the movement of labeled potassium ions in a cuttlefish axon from an external solution into the cytoplasm, (b) the rate of diffusion and the ionic mobility of the tracer along the interior of this nerve fiber, and (c) the rate of efflux from the axon to the external solution.

The results may be summarized as follows. The mixing between external and intracellular tracer potassium is a very slow process; it has a half-time of approximately 10 hr in axons 200 μ thick. If the axon behaved just like a thread of colloidal gel (e.g., agar and gelatine) 200 μ in diameter, the process of mixing should be more than half complete in seconds, not hours.

What then is the cause of this very much slower time scale? There are two possibilities: (1) potassium ions become firmly attached to internal polyelectrolytes so that their freedom of movement within the cell is greatly restricted, (2) there is a special barrier at the cell surface (the membrane), which acts as a diffusion bottleneck and restrains the mixing of otherwise freely mobile internal and external potassium ions.

The experimental procedure used by Hodgkin and Keynes was to place a small droplet of radioactive potassium on the middle portion of the isolated nerve fiber and allow a measurable quantity to enter the axoplasm. After 2 hr about 10% of the internal potassium had become labeled. The outside solution was then replaced by briefly rinsing the axon in ordinary sea water, and the real experiment commenced. The spatial "profile" of the radioactive patch along the axon was measured at intervals, and from the progressive longitudinal spread of the radioactivity the diffusion coefficient of the internal potassium ions was determined.

Secondly, a longitudinal p.d. was applied between the ends of the axon, and the velocity was determined with which the whole radioactive patch moved toward the cathode. This gave a direct measurement of the intracellular ionic mobility. Both values were only a few percent lower than the corresponding values (self-diffusion coefficient and ionic mobility) for potassium in sea water. It was clear, therefore, that the labeled ions that had entered the axoplasm continued, inside the cell, to behave as free ions with approximately normal mobility. So the slowness of the exchange between cell and surroundings cannot be explained by a restriction of ionic movement within the cell but must be due to a surface barrier.*

It is sometimes said that the phase boundary between two conducting media could itself act as a surface barrier without invoking a chemically differentiated membrane. This is true for the boundary between a polarizable metal electrode and an electrolyte solution, but it is difficult to see how this analogy can be applied to the surface of an aqueous polyelectrolyte gel surrounded by a salt solution (particularly when one is dealing with the exchange of ions, which are common to, and have similar freedom of movement in, both phases).

---

* It may be argued here that the terms "surface barrier" and "membrane" are not synonymous, but this leads merely to a semantic dispute. The word "membrane," as used by the cell physiologist, should not be taken to imply more than the postulate of a superficial layer of the cytoplasm which is chemically and physically different from the bulk of the cell interior and which endows the cell with special properties, such as excitability and the ability to maintain ionic concentration differences economically.

The conclusions drawn from the Hodgkin and Keynes experiment have been challenged on the grounds that the preliminary uptake of labeled potassium by the cell was incomplete and amounted to only about 10%. Troschin (1960) remarks that "this is the 'free potassium' fraction, which, according to the sorption theory, undergoes rapid exchange." Now Hodgkin and Keynes produced additional evidence by measuring both influx and efflux rates of tracer ions, which indicated that there were, in fact, no appreciable "inexchangeable fractions" of potassium inside the axon and that the values for the diffusion coefficient and electrophoretic mobility could be regarded as representing most or all of the intracellular potassium. But even if one were to ignore this subsidiary evidence and suppose that there are "fast" and "slow" fractions of potassium exchange, this does not alter our conclusion. For, if the freely mobile labeled ions in Hodgkin and Keynes's experiment belonged to a "fast intracellular fraction," why did it take them 2 hr to enter instead of 1 sec? The motion of this fraction was fast *inside* the cell but very slow in entering it; this brings us back to the position we started from. This presents a formidable and so far unanswered challenge to the adversaries of the membrane theory.

There are many other observations which have served to strengthen the membrane concept. Among these are the electrical measurements of the "cable constants" of nerve and muscle fibers (Cole and Hodgkin, 1939; Hodgkin and Rushton, 1946; Lorente de Nó, 1947; Katz, 1948; Falk and Fatt, 1964), which demonstrate by an entirely different method that the cytoplasm behaves as a good electrolytic conductor which is separated from the external salt solution by an insulating surface layer.

But there is an even more tangible piece of evidence which is very well known to most who have tried to dissect single muscle fibers and particularly those who have carried out some microsurgery on squid giant axons. For example, with a fairly large, 50-μ capillary that is filled with sea water or potassium-chloride solution, one can drill long channels along the axoplasm of the squid giant fiber and move the pipette about without interfering with the ability of the axon to propagate its normal impulses. As Baker, Hodgkin, and Shaw have shown, one may even with impunity squeeze most of the axoplasm out from the end and reinflate the fiber cylinder with an artificial solution of potassium salts. But as soon as one

table 1 **cable constants of nerve and muscle fibers (at about 20° C)**

FIBER	FIBER DIAMETER, μ	LENGTH CONSTANT (IN LARGE OUTSIDE VOL.), MM	TIME CONSTANT, MSEC
Squid nerve	500	5	0.7
Lobster nerve	75	2.5	2
Crab nerve	30	2.5	5
Frog muscle	75	2	24*
			(10)

* The muscle fiber has two capacitative channels which charge and discharge at different rates (Falk and Fatt, 1964). The smaller value (2.5 $\mu f/cm^2$) probably represents the capacity of the surface membrane; the more prolonged charging process may be due to the capacity of the sarcoplasmic reticulum.

locally damages the fiber surface from the inside or outside, for instance, by scraping against it or penetrating it with the same capillary, that region is irreversibly damaged. It loses its resting potential, fails to respond to stimulation, and cannot conduct impulses. It is clear that the fiber surface is the site of a specialized structure which is excitable as well as vulnerable and whose properties differ from the rest of the cell.

In order to explain why the surface membrane behaves as an ionic barrier, that is, a relative insulator between two well-conducting aqueous media, one may assume that the bulk phase of the "cellular skin" consists of fatty material, in other words, that the surface layer represents for the most part a separate lipid phase, possibly no more than a bimolecular leaflet, interposed between the cytoplasmic gel and the outside solution (see, for example, Davson and Danielli, 1943). This is the way in which measurements of alternating-current impedance of cells have been interpreted by K. S. Cole and his coworkers (1940). Furthermore, recent analyses of the cable properties of nerve and muscle fibers, which used *direct-current transients* (see Cole and Hodgkin, 1939; Hodgkin and Rushton, 1946; Lorente de Nó, 1947; Katz, 1948; Falk

MEMBRANE RESISTANCE R_m, OHM-CM^2	MEMBRANE CAPACITY C_m, μf/CM^2	RESISTIVITY OF CELL INTERIOR R_i, OHM-CM	RESISTIVITY OF MEDIUM R_o, OHM-CM
700	1	30	22
2,000	1	60	22
5,000	1	60	22
4,000	6* (2.5)	200	87

and Fatt, 1964), led researchers to the same general conclusions.

These are summarized in Table 1. The cytoplasm has a specific resistance which is between 1.5 and 3 times higher than, but remains in the same order of magnitude as, that of the external medium. The difference may be due to such factors as immobility or low mobility of some of the internal anions and the presence of nonsolvent or membrane enclosed intracellular particles that do not contribute to current flow and may present obstacles to it. Reduced activity of intracellular potassium may be another factor. (This seems to be negligible in cephalopod giant axons, but it may be more important in other fibers, particularly in muscle.)

The axon surface has a capacity of $1\mu f$/cm^2 (Cole, 1940, 1949). In many muscles, much larger values have been obtained, though there is now reason to believe that these large capacities may arise from a system of complicated tubular and reticulated channels whose surfaces are an extension of the cell membrane (Falk and Fatt, 1964). If one takes the value of $1\mu f$/cm^2 as characteristic of a lipid material that makes up the bulk of the cell membrane and assumes a dielectric constant of approximately 6, the thickness of this layer would be about 50 Å.* This material has to withstand a p.d. of roughly 0.1 volt, i.e., a field of 2×10^5 volts/cm. It is not surprising that signs of damage and dielectric breakdown begin to appear when this field is increased (by artificial hyperpolarization) by a factor of 2 to 4 (Hodgkin, 1951; del Castillo and Katz, 1954; Stämpfli, 1958).

In the electron microscope, cell membranes of various kinds have been observed (Sjöstrand, 1959; Robertson, 1960). The current view is that there are a number of adventitious connective tissue layers (collagen fibrils, basement membrane, or "ectolemma") on the outside of the actual plasmalemma which is visible as a cell border of two parallel dark lines separated by a clear space about 50 Å wide. The present-day resolution and preparatory techniques do not enable one to see any detail or differentiation in this membrane other than this double contour. One cannot be certain whether the whole of this structure is to be identified with our postulated physiological membrane. It may be that in the future, further subdivisions of the plasmalemma may appear, and one hopes that a structural differentiation will ultimately become visible within it.

The conductivity of this layer appears to be extremely low compared with that of the aqueous material on either side. Values of 1 to 10×10^{-4} ohm^{-1} cm^{-2} have usually been obtained. For a membrane 50 Å thick, this amounts to a specific resistance of the order of 10^{10} ohm cm, 100 million times greater than that of the surrounding solutions. This is a measure of the low permeability of the cell membrane to ions, even to the small ions—potassium, sodium, and chloride—which are present on either side and whose statistical chances of penetration are reduced thereby to less than 10^{-8} per individual collision.

membrane potential and ion selectivity The studies of both tracer movements and the electrical constants of the resting fiber have shown that the cell consists of a well-conducting electrolyte gel surrounded by an insulating membrane. Although the ionic permeability of this surface structure is very

* If one regards the membrane as a thin insulator between two electrolyte solutions, then its capacity per square centimeter is given by $C = 1.1 \, k / 4\pi d \times 10^{-12}$ f, where d is the thickness of the membrane and k its dielectric constant (which is a measure of the electric orientation of its molecules). For $k = 5.7$ (values for oils are usually between 2 and 7) and $C = 1\mu f/cm^2$, $d = 5 \times 10^{-7}$ cm.

low, it shows a remarkable discrimination between the different ion species. This is of great physiological importance, because the sign and size of the p.d. across the membrane is determined by its relative permeability to the principal inorganic ions, sodium, potassium, and chloride. This was recognized by Bernstein, who was the first to apply the physicochemical ideas of Nernst and Ostwald to the explanation of electrophysiological phenomena.

The basic facts and ideas from which the modern theories of bioelectricity have been developed are very simple. Electric potential differences, in general, appear at the boundaries between two electrolyte solutions if there are ions of different mobility or concentration on either side. In the absence of a membrane, one obtains a liquid-junction potential or diffusion potential. Suppose two dilute aqueous solutions of NaCl—one at a concentration (or more correctly at an average "activity") of 0.1 M and the other at 0.01 M—are making contact through a porous filter. A diffusion potential will immediately develop because Cl^- ions in aqueous solution are more mobile than Na^+ ions. Consequently, the more dilute solution will become electronegative with respect to the more concentrated side. The p.d. can be calculated from the formula

$$E = \frac{RT}{F} \frac{u - v}{u + v} \ln \frac{C_1}{C_2} = 2.3 \frac{RT}{F} \frac{u - v}{u + v} \log \frac{C_1}{C_2}$$

where R = universal gas constant

T = absolute temperature

F = "Faraday" (electric charge per gram equivalent of univalent ions)

u and v = the mobilities of Na^+ and Cl^-, respectively, along a potential gradient

C_1 and C_2 = the salt concentrations (or more correctly, the geometric mean activity of the two ions) on each side

RT/F at 20°C is approximately 25 mv; the mobility of Cl is approximately 1.5 times that of Na. Hence $(u - v)/(u + v) = -0.2$, and E is approximately -12 mv.

Suppose, however, we prevent free diffusion by placing a membrane across the boundary that is selectively permeable to the chloride ions but does not allow any sodium ions to pass. This is roughly equivalent to reducing u to zero, so we would obtain a five times larger p.d., one approximately 60 mv between the two solutions. In this case, the equation takes on the simple form of the well-known *Nernst equation*

$$E = \frac{RT}{F} \ln \frac{C_2}{C_1}$$

Let us consider another case—the boundary between aqueous solutions of NaCl and KCl of equal concentration. The mobility of potassium ions u_K is nearly the same as that of chloride v and about 50% greater than that of sodium ions u_{Na}. A diffusion potential, therefore, develops, making the KCl solution electronegative. The size of the potential difference can be derived from the equation

$$E = \frac{RT}{F} \ln \frac{u_{Na} + v}{u_K + v} = \frac{RT}{F} \ln \frac{\Lambda_1}{\Lambda_2}$$

where Λ_1/Λ_2 is the ratio of the specific conductances of the two salt solutions. The p.d. in this case amounts to approximately -5 mv.

Something should be said about the method by which the mobilities of ions in solution can be measured. The absolute mobility of an ion is defined as its average velocity of migration (cm/sec) in an electric field of 1 volt/cm. The values for K^+, Na^+, and Cl^- are included in Table 2. They are of the order of several microns per second. These values were obtained by measuring the conductivity

table 2   **mobility of some important ions***

ION	ATOMIC WEIGHT	IONIC CRYSTAL RADIUS, Å	LIMITING CONDUCT-ANCE IN H_2O†	ABSOLUTE MOBILITY IN H_2O, $(\mu/\text{SEC})/$ (VOLT/CM)	CALCU-LATED HYDRA-TION NUMBERS
Li^+	6.94	0.6	38.69	4.01	6
Na^+	23.00	0.95	50.11	5.2	4.5
K^+	39.096	1.33	73.52	7.64	2.9
Cl^-	35.46	1.81	76.34	7.91	2.9
Br^-	79.92	1.95	79.92	8.28	2.4
I^-	126.93	2.16	76.8	7.96	0

* From B. E. Conway, 1952.
† Limiting conductance is equal to equivalent conductance extrapolated for very dilute solution, in 10^3 ohm^{-1}/cm, at 25°C.

of dilute solutions of salts containing these ions and by determining the transport number (or transference number) of each ion. This is the fraction of the total current which is carried by the particular ion. It can be measured by various means, e.g., by titrating the amount which migrates to the electrode in a certain time or by observing the movement of the visible boundary between two electrolyte solutions containing a common ion.

If one compares the mobilities of the alkali metal ions Li, Na, and K, an interesting point arises. The smaller the atomic weight, the lower the ionic velocity. At first this seems strange. The smaller the size of a solute particle, whether electrically charged or neutral, the more easily one would expect it to move among the molecules of the aqueous solvent. The resistance encountered by a moving solute particle depends on friction between the solvent molecules and its own surface, and this applies to random motion by thermal agitation as well as to the directed flow in an electric field.

It may be noted in passing that the applied electric force imparts a constant average *velocity* to the ion (not constant acceleration). This is a consequence of the fact that the movement is opposed solely by frictional resistance, and the mass or the inertia of the ions can be ignored.

What, in fact, determines ionic mobility and ionic conductance is not the atomic diameter of the metal, but the size of an outer "shell" of water molecules with which the metal ion forms a complex bond and which moves with the ion through the aqueous medium. The smaller the atom inside the shell, the more strongly it "hydrates," i.e., attracts water molecules, and, therefore, the larger the cloud of water that it drags with it. This is the reason a potassium ion, in spite of the larger metal atom, can move more quickly through water than a lithium ion. Attempts have been made to calculate the size of the hydrated ion and the number of water molecules associated with it (see Table 2); for our purposes it is sufficient to note that there is an inverse relation between the velocity of an ion and the extent of its hydration or solvation.

Let us return to the discussion of the liquid junction. Suppose we place a semipermeable, porous membrane between the two solutions. The resulting p.d.'s will depend on what kind of membrane we use and on the concentrations of the ions on its two sides. We will consider three different cases (Fig. 14).

figure 14

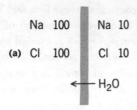

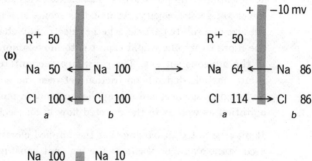

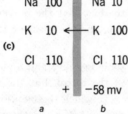

Different types of membrane and their effects on electrolyte and potential distribution. Concentrations are shown in mM/l.

(1) Suppose the membrane pores are so small that only water molecules can pass through and none of the solutes can penetrate. In this case, no ionic migration takes place and no diffusion potential will arise. If the salt concentrations are unequal on either side, water tends to move through the membrane from the more dilute to the more concentrated solution (note that the water molecules are "more concentrated" in the dilute solution). This osmotic flow of water may give rise to an electrokinetic p.d. (streaming potential); this depends on the electrostatic charge of the walls of the membrane pores and the velocity of the water flow.

(2) Suppose the membrane pores are so large that all molecules and ions of moderate size can penetrate, only large colloidal parti-

cles like proteins being excluded. In this case, diffusion will take place and liquid junction potentials will appear, whose size depends on the differential ionic mobilities within the membrane pores and on the concentrations on either side (see p. 49). The system is not in a steady state, but gradually runs down unless the concentration gradients are continuously being restored by an active "pumping" process.

The presence of charged colloidal particles on one side of the membrane would influence the final distribution of the smaller penetrating ions and under certain conditions lead to the establishment of what is called a *Donnan equilibrium*. Take the case of Fig. 14b, in which the membrane allows Na^+ and Cl^- to penetrate, but not the large cation R^+. The membrane and the walls of the compartments are supposed to be rigid structures, capable of withstanding large hydrostatic pressures. The distribution of ions at the beginning of the experiment is shown in Fig. 14b. Na^+ will diffuse from b to a, and, initially, Cl^- will go with it, although the movement of Cl^- appears to be increasingly "uphill," against a developing concentration gradient. This process will continue so long as the downhill force driving Na from b to a is greater than the opposing force driving Cl from a to b. The two forces will balance when the concentration ratios for Na and for Cl have become reciprocal, i.e., when

$$\frac{Na_a}{Na_b} = \frac{Cl_b}{Cl_a}$$

or

$$Na_a Cl_a = Na_b Cl_b$$

At this point equilibrium has been reached. The total osmotic concentration is now greater in a than in b, and the tendency of water molecules to move into a down their own concentration gradient will be balanced by the development in a of a hydrostatic pressure that is equal to the difference in osmotic pressure on the two sides.

During this equilibrated state, the tendency of Na^+ to move from b to a will be equal to that of Cl^- to move from a to b. Net movement leading to separation of these ions cannot take place; it is prevented by the development of an electrostatic p.d. across the membrane which exactly balances the concentration gradient of the diffusible ions. The p.d. is given by the Nernst formula

$$E = \frac{RT}{F} \ln \frac{Na_b}{Na_a} = \frac{RT}{F} \ln \frac{Cl_a}{Cl_b}$$

(3) The third case we want to consider is a membrane of selective ion permeability. As has already been pointed out, this will give rise to a larger p.d. than a liquid junction, because the membrane discriminates between the movements of the different ionic constituents on either side much more effectively than does the aqueous solvent in the case of a "free" boundary. To take an extreme case, suppose the membrane contains very small pores, the largest of which can accommodate hydrated potassium, but not sodium ions (which are about 50% larger). Moreover, the walls of these pores contain fixed negative charges so that only positive ions can enter and pass through them and small anions like Cl^- are excluded.

If we place unequal mixtures of NaCl and KCl solutions on either side, as in the diagram (Fig. 14c), only K ions would be able to diffuse through the membrane channels, but no migration can occur because the tendency of a small number of diffusible ions to move toward the lower concentration immediately gives rise to an electrostatic force holding them back. The presence of NaCl merely maintains osmotic equilibrium. The consequence of removing the NaCl would be the establishment of a hydrostatic pressure difference or, if the structures are not rigid, of osmotic water flow into the 0.1 M KCl compartment.

In the equilibrium condition, the p.d. would again be given by the Nernst formula (except that ion activities rather than total concentrations should be used).

$$E = \frac{RT}{F} \ln \frac{K_b}{K_a} = 60 \text{ mv approx}$$

It is fair to say that the Nernst equation is the best known and most frequently cited equation in the biological literature. The different theories of bioelectric phenomena are all based on some variant of this extremely useful formula. Its original derivation is based on simple thermodynamic principles governing the condition of electrochemical equilibrium between the *electrical work* needed to move a small quantity of ions across a boundary in one direction and the *osmotic work* needed to move the same quantity in the opposite direction.

The electrical work required to transfer 1 mole of potassium (or of any other univalent cation) against a potential difference E is EF (voltage times charge per mole of univalent ion).

The osmotic work required to move 1 mole of potassium from concentration K_a to a 10-times-higher concentration K_b can best be appreciated by considering the analogous case of work done in compressing 1 g equivalent of an ideal gas reversibly (i.e., extremely slowly and isothermally) to one-tenth of its initial volume. The gas is contained in a cylinder with a movable piston. Mechanical work W is force $\times$ distance; for a small displacement δl of the piston, the force exerted is equal to gas pressure p multiplied by cross-sectional area A of the cylinder. Hence, the work δW done is $pA\delta l$, or $p\delta v$, where v is the volume of the gas. Suppose we increase the load on the piston, i.e., the pressure, very gradually; then the work done in compressing the gas from volume v_1 to v_2 is

5 $$W = \int_{v_2}^{v_1} p \, dv$$

The gas law tells us that p and v are inversely related according to

$$pv = RT$$

Hence $p = RT/v$, and Eq. (5) can be changed to

$$W = RT \int_{v_2}^{v_1} \frac{dv}{v} = RT(\ln v_1 - \ln v_2) = RT \ln \frac{v_1}{v_2}$$

In compressing the gas, its molecules have been concentrated 10 times. Exactly the same argument can be applied to the osmotic work done in concentrating solute molecules (or "moving them from a lower to a higher concentration").

Suppose our piston were made of a rigid semipermeable membrane whose properties are those described in case 3; that is, it allows only water molecules and potassium ions to penetrate. To begin with, we have a solution of 10 mM of KCl on each side of the semi-permeable piston. We now increase the pressure very slowly, allowing time for the water molecules to escape through the piston without temperature rise and gradually concentrating the solute molecules in the cylinder. If this is done reversibly, the osmotic work will amount to

$$W = RT \ln \frac{K_2}{K_1}$$

While this proceeds, potassium ions tend to diffuse through the semipermeable piston and establish an equilibrium potential that just balances the "diffusion pressure." The equilibrium is given by equality of electrical and osmotic work, namely,

$$EF = RT \ln \frac{K_2}{K_1}$$

which brings us back to the Nernst equation.

A practical question now arises. How do we best measure such equilibrium potentials and any other kind of potential difference across semipermeable membranes? The standard procedure has been described on page 31. It makes use of a concentrated KCl solution, which forms a "bridge" between the cell interior and a reversible electrode (e.g., chloridized silver which may be dipped directly into the shank of the KCl pipette or into an intermediate salt bridge containing a Ringer/agar mixture). The purpose of using a strong KCl solution is to reduce to a minimum the inevitable diffusion potential which develops at the liquid junction between the tip of the pipette and the cytoplasm. All other electrode and junction potentials which may exist in the recording system (for instance, at the liquid junction between the large outside electrode and the Ringer's solution) are of no importance. One discards them automatically by measuring only the sudden potential change which occurs when the micropipette is inserted into the cell and again when it is withdrawn. This will give us a correct measure of the membrane potential provided that the small diffusion potential at the tip of the micropipette does not change when it is moved from the outside solution into the cytoplasm. Occasionally such changes do occur and produce erratic results. They are probably caused by a "clogging" of the tip (whose orifice is only a fraction of a micron wide) with electrically charged cell particles. It is difficult to see how the measurement of membrane potentials can be made entirely proof against such errors, but in the most carefully cross-checked experiments the results are likely to be accurate to within 1 or 2 mv.*

It is, of course, important to avoid "shunting" the cell membrane with the measuring apparatus. This would draw current from the cell and thereby disturb any existing equilibrium or steady-state condition. Furthermore, the resistance of the microelectrode tip (plus the characteristic resistance of the cell) is very high; it amounts to many megohms, and therefore the input resistance of the measuring device must be kept at many hundreds of megohms to record the full emf (electromotive force). This can be done by "backing off" the membrane potential with a potentiometer placed in series with the membrane p.d. Current flow between grid and cathode of the amplifier input can be automatically backed off by using a *cathode follower*, as described on page 16.

the Bernstein theory of bioelectric phenomena   Julius Bernstein was one of the great nineteenth-century pioneers in experimental neurophysiology. By a most ingenious mechanical method (using a ballistic galvanometer, which was connected to the tissue for brief time intervals), he was able to determine the approximate time course of an action potential long before fast recording instruments became available. In 1902 he proposed an important theory, which applied the physicochemical concepts of Nernst and Ostwald to bioelectric phenomena.

Bernstein believed that the resting cell membrane was selectively permeable to potassium alone and that this selectivity was lost during excitation, when, for a moment, numerous "pores" opened up that allowed indiscriminate penetration by other small ions, e.g., Na and Cl. There was much to commend this theory. It seemed to explain the inexpensive maintenance of the ionic concentration gradients by the resting cell, for as potassium alone tended to move down its gradient, an electrostatic force developed which opposed this tendency. The existence of the resting potential, its electric sign, and its approximate magnitude was thus explained. Bernstein's theory was also successful in predicting,

---

* Errors due to electrode junction potentials are avoided by the method of internal perfusion (Baker, Hodgkin, and Shaw, 1962), in which the cytoplasm of the squid axon is replaced by an artificial salt solution.

at least qualitatively, the lowering of the resting potential when the external potassium concentration was increased, and it took into account, in a general way, the effect of temperature on the membrane potential and the then known electrical changes during the impulse.

It took nearly 40 years before Bernstein's theory was seriously challenged. In 1939, Hodgkin and Huxley showed that excitation leads to a transient reversal, not a simple abolition, of the resting potential; this could not be explained without important modification of Bernstein's ideas. Two years later, Boyle and Conway published an important paper showing that the skeletal muscle fiber is permeable to chloride as well as potassium and that its osmotic and electrochemical behavior could be explained by the presence of a leaky membrane whose "pore sizes" admitted ions smaller than sodium. The muscle fiber seemed to follow the rules of a Donnan equilibrium, its surface membrane being, in effect, impermeable to the large organic anions synthesized inside the cell and to the external sodium ions, and the permeant ions (mostly K and Cl) distributing themselves so that $K_i/K_o = Cl_o/Cl_i$. This theory deals with many facts very successfully, but the assumption of a sodium-impermeable membrane had to be abandoned as soon as studies of tracer movements were applied to muscle tissue (Levi and Ussing, 1948; Harris and Burn, 1949; Keynes, 1954).

The experiments with radioisotopes showed, in fact, that both Na and K are in a steady state of flux across the surface membrane and that both ions are transferred at about the same rates.

This raised two important questions. First, how can we reconcile the results of the tracer experiments with our conclusions about a selective permeability, or ion conductance, of the membrane derived from electric potential measurements? Second, in view of the large force driving sodium inward (the electrochemical potential is approximately 90 mv $+ \dfrac{RT}{F} \ln \dfrac{Na_o}{Na_i} = 0.15$ volt), how does the cell maintain its ionic composition and its internal negative potential in the face of continuous exchange of all the principal small ions?

To answer the first question, let us consider the case of a single muscle fiber for which many of the relevant data have been obtained by Hodgkin and Horowicz (1959).

table 3   frog muscle fiber

	TRACER FLUX,[*] 10^{-12} MOLE/(CM^2)(SEC)	
9.2 mM Na$_i$	$\xrightarrow{\text{approx 3.5}}$ $\xleftarrow{3.5}$	120 mM Na$_o$
140 mM K$_i$	$\xrightarrow{8.8}$ $\xleftarrow{5.4}$	2.5 mM K$_o$

$E \approx -90$ mv

* Tracer-flux measurements were made on isolated muscle fibers. These were not in a perfect
steady state, for they lost about 3.4×10^{-12}
mole K/cm^2 every second (for a fiber of 100-μ
diameter, this amounts to a loss of about 3.6%
of the internal potassium store per hour).

Both Na and K ions are continuously transferred in both directions
across the cell membrane. However, the mechanism by which
individual ions are transported is not known. This is important,
because the ultimate interpretation of tracer-flux measurements
will depend very much on the underlying mechanism. It is possible,
for instance, that ions are coupled to specific carrier molecules
which allow a one-for-one exchange of Na or of K across the cell
membrane without contributing to any net movement or to electric current flow (Ussing, 1947, 1949). Such a process of coupled
"exchange diffusion" would turn up as an appreciable item in the
tracer experiments without necessarily appearing in the balance
sheet of electrical measurements at all. The point will be considered
further later on, but for the present we will make the simplest
possible assumption, that is, that the greater part of the observed
sodium and potassium fluxes is due to individual ions moving
independently of each other across the cell membrane. In other
words, we suppose tentatively that sodium and potassium migrate
through the membrane in the same way that they do in free solution. That is, their flux rates are proportional to concentration
gradients and to electric potential gradients, the main difference
being that the membrane material offers a very high resistance,
i.e., has a very low permeability to them.

This low permeability may be due to a small partition coefficient
(i.e., the ion concentration in the membrane is very low), to a
greatly reduced ionic mobility, or to both. Permeability for any
one ion species is then given by $P = (u\beta/a)(RT/F)$, where u is

electric mobility, β the partition coefficient between membrane and solution, and a the thickness of the membrane. The available data do not allow us to separate the factors u and β, but an estimate of P can be made. It should be noted that P has the physical dimension of *velocity* (cm/sec), which is also the physical dimension of ion conductance and of diffusion coefficient/thickness.

If one looks at the four components of ionic flux in Table 3, it will be apparent that the outward movement of sodium differs from the three other components in that it goes against both concentration and electric potential gradients. The efflux of sodium presents, in fact, a problem of its own. The key to this problem was found when Hodgkin and Keynes (1955) showed that the efflux of Na is due to an active process of secretion in which sodium ions are extruded from the cell at the expense of an energy-yielding metabolic reaction. The remaining ionic movements, however, are, conceivably, passive processes, and may be used tentatively as an indication of ordinary leakage of Na and K through the membrane material. We will use them, therefore, to obtain a measure of the ionic permeability.

For neutral molecules (and for ions in the absence of an electric field), permeability (cm/sec) is determined by the ratio of flux/concentration* (influx/external concentration or efflux/internal concentration). For positive ions moving *against* (from inside out) or *with* (from outside in) an electric field, the ion fluxes are not proportional to concentration alone; concentration must be multiplied by a factor that represents the effect of the electric field in lowering or raising the chances of passage of individual ions. If one makes the simplifying "constant field" assumptions used by Goldman (1943) and by Hodgkin and Katz (1949), this factor—for univalent ions—is

$$\frac{EF/RT}{1 - e^{-EF/RT}}$$

where E is potential difference across the membrane, its sign being taken as positive when the ion movement is assisted and negative when the movement is opposed by the electric field. For inward movement of Na and K, this factor is 3.7; for outward movement, it is 0.102.

---

* "Concentration" is generally used because in many cases activity coefficients are not known accurately.

We then obtain the following values for potassium permeability:

From K efflux:

$$P_K = \frac{\text{efflux}}{K_i \times 0.102} = \frac{8.8 \times 10^{-12} \text{ mole/(cm}^2)(\text{sec})}{140 \times 10^{-6} \text{ mole/cm}^3 \times 0.102}$$
$$= 6.2 \times 10^{-7} \text{ cm/sec}$$

From K influx:

$$P_K = \frac{\text{influx}}{K_o \times 3.7} = \frac{5.4 \times 10^{-12} \text{ mole/(cm}^2)(\text{sec})}{2.5 \times 10^{-6} \text{ mole/cm}^3 \times 3.7}$$
$$= 5.8 \times 10^{-7} \text{ cm/sec}$$

Thus, the values of potassium permeability obtained from influx and efflux data agree very satisfactorily.

For Na, only the influx data can be used.

$$P_{Na} = \frac{\text{influx}}{Na_o \times 3.7} = \frac{3.5 \times 10^{-12} \text{ mole/(cm}^2)(\text{sec})}{120 \times 10^{-6} \text{ mole/cm}^3 \times 3.7}$$
$$= 7.9 \times 10^{-9} \text{ cm/sec}$$

Hence the ratio between sodium and potassium permeabilities $(b = P_{Na}/P_K)$ is approximately

$$b = \frac{7.9 \times 10^{-9}}{6 \times 10^{-7}} = 0.013$$

Our first question, therefore, has been answered; the tracer-flux measurements are quite consistent with the conclusions reached from electric potential measurements, namely, that the resting cell membrane is much more (75 times more) permeable to potassium ions than to sodium ions.

The ratio b is small but not negligible. If b were zero, then the resting potential would exceed the measured value by 12 mv $(E_K = \frac{RT}{F} \ln \frac{K_o}{K_i} = -102$ mv instead of -90 mv*) and potassium

---

* The usual convention is to take the difference, inside minus outside, potential as the membrane potential. Accordingly, E_K normally has a negative sign.
Confusion sometimes arises over the use of the words "resting potential" and "action potential," which frequently refer to measured amplitudes without regard to their electric sign. Thus, if it is stated that the resting potential is "below" the potassium equilibrium level, this means simply that the value of -90 mv is *numerically* smaller than the value of -102 mv. In terms of relative levels of potential, the resting membrane potential is, of course, 12 mv less negative, i.e., it is "above" E_K.

ions would be equilibrated between cells and surroundings. In actual fact, the resting potential does not reach the potassium equilibrium level, and in these isolated muscle fibers there was a small steady net loss of potassium from the cell. Assuming that chloride ions are in equilibrium in resting muscle tissue (that is, $Cl_i/Cl_o = e^{EF/RT}$; Conway, 1957; Hodgkin, 1958), then the observed resting potential E can be calculated from the data in Table 3 by the following equation (Hodgkin, 1958)

6
$$E = \frac{RT}{F} \ln \frac{K_o + bNa_o}{K_i + bNa_i} = 58 \text{ mv} \log \frac{2.5 + 0.013 \times 120}{140 + 0.013 \times 9.2} = -89 \text{ mv}$$

which agrees well with the observed value of -90 mv.

Conversely, if one derives the permeability ratio b from the observed value E and Eq. (6), b is found to agree closely with that obtained from tracer-flux measurements. With this low value of b, Eq. (6) also fits the observation, known since Bernstein's experiments and studied quantitatively by R. H. Adrian (1956), that the resting potential can be reduced very effectively if the external potassium is increased but is hardly reduced at all if the external sodium concentration is raised.

So far, the theoretical treatment of the electrical and the chemical tracer data from muscle fibers has been successful and given mutually consistent results. Nevertheless, there is evidence that the underlying assumption, namely independent migration of Na and K ions through the membrane, is oversimplified. It does not apply to all tissues, and even in muscle fibers it is probable that a substantial part of the Na and K flux occurs by more complicated mechanisms in which the transfer or exchange of ions across the membrane does not proceed independently, but by a specific mutual coupling.

It has already been pointed out that obvious inconsistencies would arise if one were to try and apply our permeability formula to the efflux of sodium. In this case "P_{Na}" would be

$$\frac{\text{Efflux}}{Na_i \times 0.102} \approx \frac{3.5 \times 10^{-12} \text{ mole}/(\text{cm}^2)(\text{sec})}{9.2 \times 10^{-6} \text{ mole/cm}^3 \times 0.102}$$
$$\approx 3.7 \times 10^{-6} \text{ cm/sec}$$

Thus, one would obtain the paradoxical result that the outward permeability for sodium is nearly 500 times greater than the inward permeability. This result merely illustrates that the assumption of independent ion migration, subject to electrical and concentration gradients, does not apply to the efflux of sodium, which goes uphill against both gradients. Either Na ions are actively extruded from the cell, so as to balance the rate at which they leak inward, or neither inward nor outward movements of Na obey the laws of independent ion movement, but are tightly coupled together by a process called *exchange diffusion*. These possibilities do not exclude each other, but at present the evidence for the second mechanism is rather scant and less compelling than that for an active sodium-extruding "pump."

During their study of cephalopod axons, Hodgkin and Keynes found that even the measurements of potassium flux were inconsistent with the theory of independent ionic migration. Part of the inward movement of potassium was dependent on the metabolism of the cell and closely linked to the active sodium efflux. The remainder of the potassium flux was passive and was directly related to the electric field and potassium concentration gradient. But there was evidence for mutual interference between inward and outward movement, as though the potassium ions were constrained to move in single file through narrow channels (or in a series of steps along a chain of reactive sites).

Suppose the membrane channels are little wider than the hydrated K ion itself and their length is taken up by a row of three or four ions. If a labeled ion happens to enter the channel from the outside, by random collision, the row of ions is displaced and, probably, one ion is released into the cytoplasm. The result is a net transfer of one ion from the outside to the interior of the cell, without entry of the labeled ion. If the next collision comes from the other direction, the labeled ion may be ejected and return to the external medium; hence, its chances of continuing to move forward in three or four successive steps are small. Its chance of penetration, however, is greatly increased if an additional electric field is applied that assists each forward push and opposes the backward step. In a system of this kind, there is an apparent discrepancy between electrically measured K conductance and diffusional tracer flux. The conductance is three to four times larger than would be predicted from the tracer flux for a membrane in which individual ions move independently (Hodgkin and Keynes, 1955*b*).

A good deal of criticism has been directed against the membrane concept on the basis of the kinetics of tracer- or chemical-flux data. Their time course does not in general follow a simple exponential curve, which is what one would expect on a simple "two compartment" hypothesis (outside solution-membrane-cell interior). To explain such departures from first-order kinetics, it has been proposed that the intracellular ion content is divided into two or more fractions or cell compartments of different degrees of "exchangeability." It must be admitted that the picture of two simple compartments, cellular and extracellular, separated by a resistive membrane is oversimplified and in many instances does not really correspond to the experimental situation. For example, the presence of adventitious tissue (e.g., a Schwann-cell layer around the giant axon) and of membrane-bound intracellular particles (mitochondria, nuclei, endoplasmic reticulum) could present a significant complicating feature even when one is working on a single nerve or muscle fiber. If one uses whole tissue, e.g., a muscle composed of hundreds of fibers of varying diameters, additional complications arise because one may be dealing with a nonuniform population of cells whose equilibration times vary over a wide range. All one can say at present is that a convincing interpretation of kinetic-flux measurements has been achieved only in rare instances and that departures from first-order kinetics are not unexpected and cannot themselves be taken as contrary to the membrane concept outlined above.

the sodium pump Perhaps the most revealing result of tracer studies on resting nerve cells was the finding by Hodgkin and Keynes (1955a) that the uphill movement of sodium from the cytoplasm to the outside can be switched off reversibly by the use of metabolic inhibitors (dinitrophenol, azide, cyanide). The pumping process can then be started up again by intracellular injection of specific energy-yielding substrates [adenosine triphosphate (ATP) and arginine phosphate; see Caldwell et al., 1960]. These observations were made on isolated cephalopod axons; the situation in muscle is less clear, and the importance of resting metabolism in pumping sodium out of muscle fibers is still a controversial matter. Ling (1962) denies it, and Steinbach (1940), Desmedt (1953), Keynes and Maisel (1954), Conway et al. (1961), and Dee and Kernan (1963) have obtained positive evidence for it.

In the nerve axon, it is certain that the efflux of sodium is controlled by an energy-yielding metabolic reaction in which the breakdown of ATP plays an important part. Another finding of great significance was that only the efflux of (labeled) sodium ions was affected by the inhibitors; the influx, proceeding downhill and requiring no energy expenditure, showed little or no change.

This provides a general answer to our question regarding maintenance of ionic composition (p. 58). The steady state of the resting cell and its large electrochemical potential gradients are maintained at the expense of a continuous "basal metabolism." This provides free energy that is utilized, in some unknown way, to expel sodium ions from the cell as fast as they are able to enter through the slightly leaky cell membrane.

The detailed mechanism of the sodium pump is still far from clear. A number of interesting questions have been posed to which so far only incomplete answers are available.

The first question is: does the pump act as a direct source of current, separating sodium from other ions and transferring positive charges outward? This would represent a "fuel cell" in which a chemical reaction directly generates an emf across the cell membrane and causes other diffusible ions like potassium and chloride to distribute themselves between inside and outside, according to their electric charge, until their concentrations are in equilibrium with the emf. The steady state of this system would be preserved so long as the cell maintains its internal concentration of indiffusible anions and actively extrudes sodium.

Alternatively, the secretion of sodium might be an electrically neutral process. This would be the case if the outward transfer of an Na ion requires an obligatory anion to go with it or if the pump works as a cation exchanger in which the outward movement of each Na ion is coupled with the inward movement of a K ion. The development of a p.d. would be an indirect effect, resulting from accumulation of potassium inside the cell and from the differential permeability of the membrane to sodium and potassium ions (p. 61).

There are at present various lines of evidence, some favoring the idea of a "concentration" pump and others that of a direct "potential" pump. It may well be that we are dealing here not with alternative processes, but with a mechanism that contains some of the features of each.

In experiments on frog nerves, Connelly (1959) has found that under certain conditions, when the uphill movement of sodium is proceeding at a particularly high rate, the membrane potential apparently rises well above the potassium equilibrium level. These observations are difficult to explain unless the efflux of sodium can contribute directly to the emf at the fiber surface.

On the other hand, in experiments on cephalopod axons, Hodgkin and Keynes showed that the extrusion of sodium can be virtually stopped by the use of metabolic inhibitors without any immediate effect on the resting potential. There ensues a slow progressive decline of the emf, but this is merely the consequence of gradual unchecked mixing of Na and K, which results in a slow decline of the ionic concentration gradients. Clearly, the activity of the sodium pump makes little or no direct contribution to the resting emf in these nerves. Furthermore, the rate of Na extrusion was found to be unaltered when the resting potential was increased by 40 mv. The efflux was, however, closely related to the concentration of Na ions inside the cell. It appears that the activity of the pump is automatically regulated by any departure of the internal Na concentration from the low level that it is designed to maintain.

The idea of a specific Na/K exchange pump received strong support when it was found that the same metabolic poisons which inhibit the efflux of Na also reduce the *inward* movement (not the efflux) of K ions. Furthermore, Hodgkin and Keynes (1955a) showed that a large part of the active extrusion of Na ceases when K ions are removed from the external medium. The natural inference from these experiments is that both the accumulation of K as well as the extrusion of Na by the cell are brought about to a large extent by a single, coupled transport mechanism (Fig. 15). The molecular forces by which a metabolic reaction (involving probably the breakdown of ATP) is geared to the specific process of ion secretion remain unknown. An interesting start has been made toward the solution of this problem with the discovery that the membranes of hemolyzed and "reconstituted" red blood cells (red cell "ghosts") contain an enzyme which hydrolyzes ATP and which possesses some of the characteristic "directional" prop-

figure 15

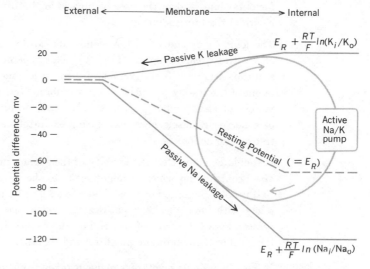

Electrochemical (downhill) gradients and ionic (uphill) pumps. Electrochemical potential differences cause K to leak outward and Na to leak inward through the cell membrane. Ionic distribution is maintained by an active secretory process, requiring continuous supply of energy. (Note: The *electric* potential gradient across the membrane is indicated by the broken line.)

cities one would ascribe to an agent responsible for active ion transport. Not only is this ATPase located in the cell surface, but it was found to be activated by external potassium and internal sodium (Glynn, 1962). Furthermore, it is inhibited by low concentrations of cardiac glycosides (e.g., ouabain or digoxin) which are known to be potent inhibitors of the uphill transport of Na and K in nerve and muscle (Post, et al., 1960; Dunham and Glynn, 1961; see also Schatzmann, 1953, Skou, 1957, and Whittam, 1958).

To summarize this chapter, we may say that the steady state of the axon, that is, the unequal distribution of ions and the maintenance of the p.d., depends on the utilization of the metabolic energy supplied by the cell for the purpose of simultaneously expelling sodium which has leaked into the cell and helping to accumulate potassium in the interior. The primary result is the building up and maintenance of large ionic concentration gradients across the surface membrane. The maintenance of the resting potential is a secondary consequence of this; it results from the fact that the resting axon membrane has a much higher conductance for potassium (and in the case of muscle for both potassium and chloride) than for sodium.

The ionic conductances of the membrane can be represented by an electric circuit diagram (Fig. 16). This type of circuit representation has been found very useful in explaining not only the origin of the resting potential of the membrane but also the great variety of electric changes which take place during the activity of a nerve or muscle fiber and during excitatory and inhibitory transmitter actions at synapses.

It should be noted that the activity of the sodium pump (and any *direct* contribution which it might make to the membrane potential) is not represented in this scheme (see Fig. 15). It is concerned solely with ionic "leakage pathways," which, according to our present knowledge, are of overriding importance in determining the level of the membrane potential and its rapid changes.

ionic equilibrium potential, ionic conductance, and membrane potential

In Fig. 16, a single membrane element taken from the cable structure of Fig. 11 is shown in detail. The diagram shows three separate conducting channels corresponding to the three prevalent inorganic ions. It indicates that the membrane has a leakage resistance to each of them and that these resistances are subject to independent physiological variation, as will become evident later on. Each channel has a characteristic electromotive force which is known as the *equilibrium potential* for the particular ion. This emf represents

figure 16

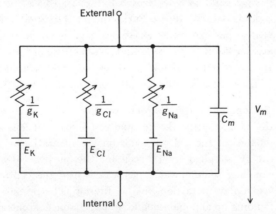

Equivalent electric circuit diagram of nerve or muscle membrane. $E_K = -70$ to -100 mv (inside negative); $E_{Na} = +50$ to $+65$ mv; $E_{Cl} = -45$ to -90 mv. (Modified from Hodgkin, 1958.)

the electrical p.d. across the membrane that would just balance the tendency of the ion to diffuse in the direction of its concentration (or rather of its chemical activity) gradient. Thus, for positive ions like K and Na, the electric polarity is opposite to the concentration difference. For chloride, electric polarity and concentration gradient have the same direction. The size of the emf is given by the Nernst equation, that is, $E_{Na} = \dfrac{RT}{F} \ln (Na_o/Na_i)$. (The convention regarding electrical sign is to have zero potential, i.e., the reference level, in the external fluid. The interior of the resting cell is at a *negative* potential, the p.d. across the resting membrane being taken as $V_i - V_o$.)*

The actual value of the p.d. across the membrane (in the absence of an applied emf or of an electrical pump) must lie somewhere between the extreme values given by the equilibrium potentials for sodium and potassium. If one of the ionic conductances predominates, the membrane potential will move close to the emf of this particular channel.

Suppose that as the result of a chemical action or some other disturbance the conductance of one channel (e.g., sodium) increases temporarily by an amount Δg_{Na}. This causes an extra flow of current $(E_{Na} - V_m) \Delta g_{Na}$. The current flow alters the charge on the membrane capacity and displaces V_m toward E_{Na} [the initial value of $dV/dt = (E_{Na} - V_m) \times \Delta g_{Na}/C$]. It will be apparent that a knowledge of the equilibrium potentials has some diagnostic value in determining the nature of a transient permeability change. If we artificially displace V_m by various amounts, for instance, by passing steady currents of varying intensities through the membrane, a null point will be found beyond which the effects of Δg, that is, the extra flow of current and the direction of the potential change, reverse their signs (Fig. 17). In our example, this reversal point will be reached when $V_m = E_{Na}$, and in general this simple null point method may enable one to decide whether a specific ionic gate is being opened up during a physiological reaction.

In muscle the normal resting potential is very close to, possibly identical with, E_{Cl} (Hodgkin, 1958); this suggests that chloride ions

---

* Unless these conventions are kept in mind, confusion might arise over the terminology; for example, when the *internal potential* is raised (made less negative), the p.d. *across the membrane* becomes less and the membrane is said to become depolarized.

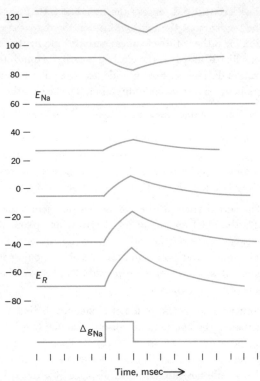

figure 17

Change of potential V_m in model membrane (Fig. 16) resulting from a brief increase of Na permeability (Δg_{Na}) of fixed magnitude. E_R = resting potential; E_{Na} = Na-equilibrium level. The initial levels of V_m have been adjusted by passing steady outward currents of different intensities through the membrane. (Note: In constructing this diagram, it has been assumed for simplicity that apart from Δg_{Na} no subsequent alterations of ion permeability occur when the membrane potential changes. In most nerve and muscle cells this assumption does not hold; the actual effect is then more complicated because depolarization would lead to further permeability changes and the initiation of action potentials.)

distribute themselves passively until their concentration gradient is in equilibrium with the potential gradient. Potassium ions are nearly, but not quite, equilibrated: the resting p.d. is somewhat below the level at which a net loss of potassium ions down their concentration gradient would be prevented. Sodium ions are very far from their electrochemical equilibrium. So the result is that in the system shown in Fig. 16, a steady circulating current flows outward through the potassium channel (K ions leaking out of the cell) and inward through the sodium channel (Na ions entering the cell), the two ionic leakage rates being equal in intensity and opposite in sign. The resting potential is much closer to E_K than to E_{Na}; this is so because the permeability and ionic conductance to sodium are much lower than to potassium. To maintain the system in a steady state, the Na and K batteries (depending on the concentration differences of these ions) must be recharged. This is done continuously by the ionic pump mentioned on p. 64 (not represented in Fig. 16), which in turn derives its energy from organic phosphate metabolism. We have then a coupling of two distinct processes: a continuous expenditure of metabolic energy which serves to replenish an ionic reservoir. This latter presents a ready store of electrochemical energy on which the nerve cell can draw during periods of intense signaling activity.

The scheme of Fig. 16 formally indicates that rapid changes of the membrane potential, for instance, those which occur during the impulse or synaptic activation, arise from changes in ionic conductance and not from alterations of the ionic emf. The latter depends on internal and external ion concentrations which would, under physiological conditions, only change very slowly. It should be noted, however, that this is a simplified scheme. It can be used to explain rapid electric alterations, but does not necessarily apply to slow cumulative potential changes during long trains of impulses (afterpotentials). These may well depend on a gradual change of the ion content of the cell (especially in fibers of small diameter and low volume/surface ratio) or of the immediate surroundings (especially if there are diffusion "bottlenecks," e.g., connective tissue layers, Schwann cells, etc., between them and the main external volume). Such cases have been discussed in detail by Frankenhaeuser and Hodgkin, 1956, and Ritchie and Straub, 1957.

Another important point which sometimes gives rise to confusion is explained very simply by the scheme in Fig. 16. It is common experience in the study of "synaptic potentials" that small potential changes of the same kind are produced in an effector cell (e.g., motor neuron or muscle end plate) by the activity of many individual nerve endings or even smaller presynaptic "units" (see p. 131). Within certain limits, such small potentials are all *additive*, although they occur in *parallel* at many neighboring spots of the same postsynaptic cell membrane. The reasons are, of course, that each of the individual potential changes is the result of a small increment in membrane conductance and that similar parallel conductance changes are additive and produce additional ionic current.

ionic conductance and ion permeability

The terms "ionic conductance" and "ionic permeability" are often used as though they are interchangeable, but this is not, in fact, the case, though permeability P as defined on p. 60 happens to have the same dimension as that of a conductance (cm/sec). It is true that the two properties are intimately related and, in practice, *rapid changes* of one quantity are usually concurrent with similar changes in the other. On the "constant field" theory of Goldman (1943), and Hodgkin and Katz (1949), the relation between potassium permeability P_K and membrane conductance g_K (ohm^{-1} cm^{-2}) for very small potassium current is given by

$$g_K = \frac{P_K F^3 E K_0}{R^2 T^2 \left(e^{EF/RT} - 1\right)}$$

where E is the membrane p.d. and K_o is the external potassium concentration. The potassium conductance is not a simple constant: it depends not only on the potassium permeability P_K but also on the number and distribution of potassium ions available on either side and within the membrane. The physical difference between conductance and permeability may be visualized if we think of a foreign anion A^-, which is not normally present and so contributes nothing to normal membrane conductance but for which the membrane has a very high permeability—$P_A \gg P_K$, P_{Cl}. If we were to replace external chloride by this foreign anion, the membrane conductance would greatly increase, although no permeability change would take place.

5

the initiation of the impulse

two factors
in the
propagation of
an impulse:
cable
conduction
and
excitation

Nerve and muscle fibers are cylindrical conductors surrounded by surface membranes, which insulate them from the external electrolyte solution. This endows the fibers with properties analogous to those of a submarine cable. Characteristic cable constants have been listed in Table 1 (p. 47). Now it is clear that, quantitatively, this analogy cannot be pursued very far. The conductance of the core, a thin thread of electrolytic gel, is many million times lower than that of the metallic core of a long-distance submarine cable, and the insulation of the sheath, millimicrons instead of millimeters thick, is similarly inferior. The result is that a brief subthreshold signal cannot travel more than a millimeter or two along a fiber without becoming grossly distorted and attenuated because of capacitative and resistive leakages through the surface membrane and because of energy dissipation in the fiber core.

This point may be appreciated most easily if one considers the losses due to the resistance of the axoplasm and the leakage conductance of the membrane (Fig. 18). For an axon immersed in a large volume of conducting fluid, the outside resistance may be ignored and the external potential regarded as constant. The internal resistance per unit length is r_i (ohm/cm) and the conductance of the membrane per unit length is $1/r_m$ (ohm^{-1}/cm). Suppose a signal of amplitude V_0 (p.d. across membrane) has been applied at one point of the axon. Its forward spread depends on the amount of longitudinal current which flows along the core. This is

7 $\quad i_{\text{long}} = -\dfrac{1}{r_i}\dfrac{dV}{dx} \quad$ [cf. Eq. (2)]

The longitudinal current diminishes with increasing distance x because part of it leaks away to the outside through the membrane conductance. This part is the membrane current i_m. Hence

figure 18

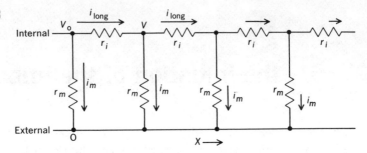

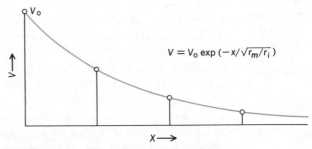

$$V = V_0 \exp\left(-x/\sqrt{r_m/r_i}\right)$$

Spread of voltage and current along a resistive cable. r_m = radial membrane resistance × cm; r_i = longitudinal core resistance/cm. The "length constant" of the cable is $\sqrt{r_m/r_i}$.

8 $$-\frac{di_{long}}{dx} = i_m = \frac{V}{r_m}$$

From Eqs. (7) and (8)

$$\frac{r_m}{r_i}\frac{d^2V}{dx^2} = V$$

The solution of this differential equation is

$$V = A \exp\left(\frac{-x}{\sqrt{r_m/r_i}}\right) + B \exp\left(\frac{+x}{\sqrt{r_m/r_i}}\right)$$

Since $V = 0$ at $x = \infty$, $B = 0$. If $V = V_0$ at $x = 0$, the particular solution is

$$V = V_0 \exp\left(\frac{-x}{\sqrt{r_m/r_i}}\right)$$

Hence, the voltage signal fades out in exponential fashion with increasing distance x, falling to $1/e$ with a length constant $\sqrt{r_m/r_i}$. As expected, the higher the membrane resistance and the lower the resistance of the core, the further the signal spreads. The values of r_m and r_i vary inversely with the size of the fiber. Their relation to the *specific* resistances of one cm² of membrane R_m and one cm³ of axoplasm R_i is given by

$$r_m = \frac{R_m}{2\pi\rho}$$

$$r_i = \frac{R_i}{\pi\rho^2}$$

where ρ is the fiber radius. Hence, the length constant is $\sqrt{\rho R_m/2R_i}$; that is, it varies with the square root of the fiber size. For example, a nonmyelinated crustacean axon of 30-μ diameter with values of $R_m = 5{,}000$ ohm-cm² and $R_i = 50$ ohm-cm has a length constant of 2.7 mm. With brief pulses, the attenuation of the signal is much more severe because most of the current is shunted through the membrane capacity.

In spite of all these defects, the continuous cable linkage between one region of a fiber and the next is an indispensable factor in passing on electrical changes from point to point. This was first suggested by Hermann's local-circuit theory and has been established experimentally by Hodgkin (1937). See also Makarov and Judenich, 1929; Lillie, 1936; Lorente de Nó, 1947; and Tasaki, 1939, 1953.

Furthermore, it can fairly be said that the cable properties of the neuron are the physical basis for all integrative processes at central nervous synapses. For example, spatial summation (or subtraction) of synaptic effects that interact within an effector cell depend upon the spread of subthreshold electric signals along the cell membrane. And as the synapses are clustered closely together within a fraction of a millimeter of the cell body, local integration of such signals can be handled by the subthreshold cable properties of the membrane. An entirely different problem, however, is the analysis of the mechanism by which the afferent impulses arriving in presynaptic nerve terminals are able to impress local signals on the surface of the effector cell. For the two cells are separated by their membranes and by a small extracellular gap, and this structural discontinuity—as we shall see in more detail later—appears in many cases to rule out any possibility of cable connection between one neuron and the next. It seems that the core conductor, or cable mechanism, is not involved in the transmission of signals *across* most synapses, although it undoubtedly is the basis for the *integration* of local messages once these have been transferred to the common effector cell.

With regard to the peripheral axon, or muscle fiber, the problem we want to consider is how the cell makes up for the defects of its cable properties and ensures that a signal is conveyed over long distances without attenuation. An important clue to this problem was provided when the initiation of an impulse with a brief electric current was studied. The experimental procedure is much the same as that shown in Fig. 10. When a short current pulse is passed inward through the fiber membrane, the membrane potential is displaced. The surface capacity is charged up to a higher p.d.; this rapidly falls again after the end of the pulse to the steady initial level of the membrane potential. When the direction of the current pulse is reversed, we obtain a similar picture of opposite polarity provided the current intensity is weak. But as the membrane p.d. is lowered from its normal value of 70 to 90 mv to about 60 mv or slightly less, the observed effect changes. The displacement of the membrane potential increases out of proportion to the applied current strength, and at the end of the pulse, the recovery of the initial resting potential is somewhat delayed. With a slight further increase of current intensity, this phenomenon becomes much more pronounced, and a critical level is reached at which the membrane potential—if left to itself—lingers for a variable time and then either flares up into a propagating spike or simply returns to the baseline. The family of curves shown in Fig. 19 is very characteristic of the local events which lead to a propagated impulse in all excitable tissues, and it has been pointed out repeatedly that similar behavior can be obtained from a large variety of inanimate physical or chemical systems which have the ingredients required for a regenerative chain reaction.

In the present case, a lowering of membrane potential, if it is driven beyond a certain unstable point (the threshold), leads to an auto-

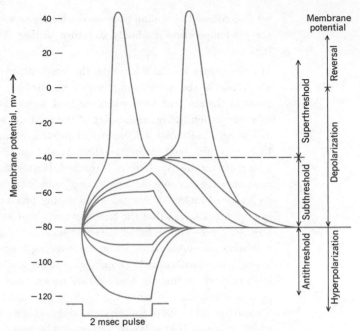

The initiation of an impulse by local depolarization. Current pulses of fixed duration (indicated below) but variable size and polarity cause variations of membrane potential shown by the family of curves (above).

matic transient reinforcement of the initial displacement (the spike). But one could obtain a family of curves similar to that shown in Fig. 19 by using an explosive gas mixture, say hydrogen and oxygen, and by plotting the temperature of the gas (instead of the height of the membrane potential) against a suitable time scale. The stimulus for our gas mixture would be the application of heat (instead of electric current).

Consider first the downward displacement of the system away from its firing point. We do this by cooling, i.e., by withdrawing heat at a constant rate. The temperature of the mixture falls below the stable level of the surroundings, and unless the gas is perfectly insulated, heat will flow into it from the environment. The rate of cooling, therefore, gradually diminishes until equilibrium is reached at a lower temperature (when the rate of heat withdrawal is balanced by the rate of leakage from the warmer surroundings). When we discontinue the cooling process, the leakage goes on and causes the gas temperature gradually to return to that of the surroundings.

When we *apply* heat at a low rate, the temperature of the gas rises above that of the surroundings with a similar time course and returns to the ambient level when the heat supply is stopped. But as we approach the ignition point of the mixture, some hydrogen and oxygen molecules will react and produce extra heat tending to increase the temperature further. At the ignition point itself, a level of unstable equilibrium is reached. If we withdraw our heat appliance, the gas goes on "smoldering" and for an uncertain time its scattered molecular reactions will supply just as much heat as is lost by leakage, so that the temperature is kept at a precariously unstable level—above that of the environment. A slight diminution will bring the system back to the surrounding temperature, and a slight increase will cause the combustion to become self-reinforcing and explosive, so that the temperature rises rapidly to a very high peak and only returns when the mixture is completely burnt out. We can see the limits of this crude analogy. It is a "kinetic" model which indicates that a family of curves like that in Fig. 19, displaying three different regions (antithreshold, subthreshold, and superthreshold), can be obtained from any explosive reaction. But it tells us nothing direct about the physical chemistry underlying nerve excitation, and if taken too far, the analogy becomes misleading. It is clear, for instance, that the passage of an impulse leaves the nerve fiber, unlike our gas mixture, quite unexhausted and ready to repeat the event many times, at intervals of 1 or 2 msec.

The question thus remains: what is the nature of the regenerative process by which a partial depolarization of the membrane potential becomes amplified automatically? The answer was found during a series of experiments on the squid giant axon (Hodgkin, 1958) in which it was shown that the sodium conductance g_{Na} is a function of the membrane potential. At the normal resting potential g_{Na} is very small, but it increases when the resting potential is lowered. We do not yet know *why* this happens, but it is a fact of greatest importance. For as a consequence, sodium ions will enter the fiber at an increased rate and, by carrying their positive charge across the membrane, will reinforce the initial lowering of the resting potential (Fig. 20). This in turn causes the Na permeability

figure 20

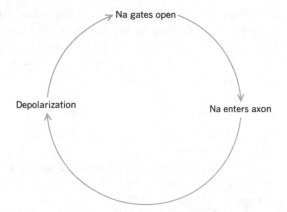

Na gates open

Depolarization

Na enters axon

Diagram showing the mutual reinforcement of membrane depolarization and sodium permeability increase.

to rise; thus the process can become "explosive." It is worth noting that the extra Na current takes place in spite of a positive potential increment of the fiber interior, that is, in opposition to Ohm's law. In other words, because of its characteristic permeability change, the membrane offers a "negative resistance" to sodium ions over a certain range of its voltage/current relation.

Returning for a moment to our explosive-gas analogy, we see that the *regenerative* factor in the axon membrane (corresponding to the exothermic combination of the gas molecules) is the increase of sodium conductance. The *restoring* factor (which corresponds to the loss of heat by leakage) is the conductance of the potassium and chloride channels which tends to return the displaced potential toward its original level. The "ignition point" of the system (threshold potential) is reached when, after the withdrawal of the current pulse, the rate of sodium entry is sufficiently high to balance the simultaneous potassium efflux and chloride influx and so maintain the depolarization in an unstable equilibrium. A slight decrease in the sodium current will cause the activity to die out (this is the local, or subthreshold, response); a slight increase in the inward current of sodium will cause the potential change and the coupled increase of Na conductance to flare up rapidly and displace the membrane potential toward the sodium equilibrium level E_{Na} (Figs. 16 and 19). Theoretically, therefore, the sodium entry could continue to overpower all other ion movements until the cytoplasm acquires sufficient positive potential (about +50 to +60 mv relative to the outside) to balance the chemical potential gradient of Na ions. In practice, this level is never quite attained during the course of an action potential because (1) the opening of the Na gates is only a brief transient event and (2) it is rapidly followed by an increase in the K conductance, which begins to operate near the peak of the action potential and accelerates the return of the system to its resting condition.

This is a brief summary of the conclusions which resulted from a series of striking experiments by A. L. Hodgkin, A. F. Huxley, and their colleagues (Hodgkin and Huxley, 1952a). That sodium ions play a key role during electric excitation was first indicated by the experiments of Overton (1902) at the beginning of this century, who showed that the excitability of muscle depends specifically on the presence of sodium in the environment and who went so far as to suggest that an exchange between Na and K across the cell membrane might be the source of the electric currents generated during nerve and muscle activity. That excitation depends on an increase of membrane permeability had also been foreseen long ago by Bernstein, who thought of it in terms of a general breakdown of an ionic barrier. This view received strong evidence from the experiments of Cole and Curtis (1939), who showed that a striking increase of ion conductance accompanies the passage of a nerve impulse. When the presence of graded subthreshold responses and their gradual transition into an impulse was discovered (Rushton, 1932; Auger and Fessard, 1935; Katz, 1937, 1947; Hodgkin, 1938; Rosenblueth, 1952; del Castillo and Stark, 1952), it became clear that a regenerative factor was involved and that membrane excitation depends probably on a negative resistance to some species or combination of ions. Hodgkin and Huxley (1939) and Cole and Curtis (1942) observed that the action potential is not a wave of *depolarization* (which was the basis of Bernstein's hypothesis) but of transient *reversal* of the resting potential; this finding pointed to a reversal of the characteristic ion selectivity (i.e., the ratio P_{Na}/P_K) of the membrane. This avenue of thought was then carefully explored (Hodgkin and Katz, 1949; Nastuk and Hodgkin, 1950; Hodgkin, Huxley, and Katz, 1949, 1952; Hodgkin and Huxley, 1952a to 1952e; Keynes, 1951; Keynes and Lewis, 1951; Huxley and Stämpfli, 1950; and Frankenhaeuser, 1960) in a series of investigations on various types of nerve and muscle fibers.

In all these instances, excitability was quickly and reversibly abolished when sodium was withdrawn from the external medium. Unlike the resting potential (which is potassium-dependent but not sodium-dependent), the membrane p.d. at the crest of the action potential and the steepest rate of ascent of the spike are directly related to the external sodium concentration.

The ionic theory of the action potential enables one to predict the minimum quantity of sodium ions that must enter the axon during the rising phase of the wave and the equivalent amount of potassium that must leave by exchange during the falling phase. These quantities are simply the electrochemical equivalent of the coulombs needed to displace the membrane potential from the resting level to the top of the spike and back again; i.e., approximately 0.1 volt $\times$ 1 $\mu f/(cm^2)$(faraday) = 10^{-12} moles/cm^2 both ways. This represents net positive charge transferred; in practice, a larger quantity of sodium must enter during the rising phase in order to balance the growing countercurrent of potassium ions.

These predictions were tested in tracer-flux experiments (Keynes, 1951; Keynes and Lewis, 1951) in which the rates of ion movements were compared during periods of rest and prolonged impulse activity. Furthermore, by an ingenious application of radioactivation analysis (isolated nerve fibers which had either been resting or conducting many impulses were subjected to neutron bombardment and their radioactive Na and K contents were determined), changes of cellular sodium and potassium levels could be measured. Finally, with the help of fine Na- and K-selective glass microelectrodes, Hinke (1961) was able to observe the changes in intracellular cation activity resulting from a train of impulses. These different techniques produced a very consistent answer, namely, that a giant axon takes up 3 to 4 $\times$ 10^{-12} mole Na/cm^2 and loses the same amount of potassium per impulse. Thus, there is no doubt that the total quantity of sodium which enters the fiber is more than sufficient to provide the necessary electric current for the nerve signal.

The evidence for the sodium theory was greatly strengthened by applying the method of voltage control [or voltage clamp (Fig. 21); see Cole, 1949; Hodgkin, Huxley and Katz, 1949]. This technique enables one to prevent the automatic and explosive development of the spike and to change the membrane potential in controlled

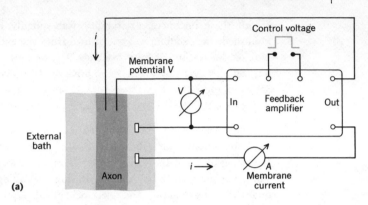

(a)

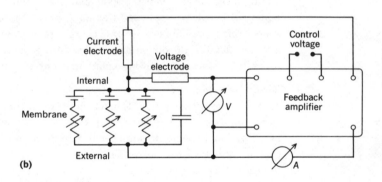

(b)

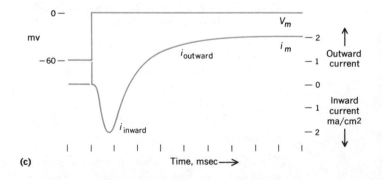

(c)

Diagram of ''voltage clamp'' (a and b) and of the measurement of membrane current during voltage displacement (c).

steps. In order to do this, a feedback amplifier is connected to two electrodes on either side of the membrane and automatically supplies the current needed to shift the membrane potential and maintain it at any desired level.

For example, the membrane can be suddenly and completely depolarized; that is, its p.d. is dropped from the normal resting level to zero (Fig. 22). The associated current flow has three discrete components. First, there is a momentary surge of *outward* current due to the discharge of the membrane capacity, approximately 6×10^{-8} coul/cm^2 being withdrawn within a few microseconds. After this initial displacement current, the membrane capacity remains completely discharged and the subsequent current flow must, therefore, be attributed to ions passing through the conductance channels of the membrane. The second phase is a surge of *inward* current, that is, cations entering, or anions emerging from, the axoplasm, reaching a peak value of several ma/cm^2. It should be noted that the direction of this component of current is in opposition to Ohm's law (positive current flows into the axon, although the potential of the interior has been stepped up from -60 mv to 0). This phase is again a transient phenomenon in spite of maintained depolarization; within 1 or 2 msec it is converted into a phase of persistent outward current which continues to flow at an intensity of several ma/cm^2 for as long as the depolarized state of the membrane is kept up. This final outward current follows Ohm's law, but its intensity is very high, which indicates that the membrane resistance has fallen to a low value. The nature of the third component has been clarified by Hodgkin and Huxley, who showed in tracer measurements that the whole of the maintained outward current is accounted for by an electrochemically equivalent efflux of potassium ions from the axoplasm. It appeared therefore that a delayed, but maintained, result of depolarization is a large increase in the potassium permeability.

The nature of the transient inward current was elucidated by determining its null point, i.e., by finding the membrane p.d. at which the direction of this component just reverses sign. This "equilibrium level" was reached when $E = \dfrac{RT}{F} \ln \dfrac{\mathrm{Na}_o}{\mathrm{Na}_i}$. Normally E is approximately 50 mv (positive inside), which is not far from the peak value of the action potential. If the external Na concentra-

figure 22

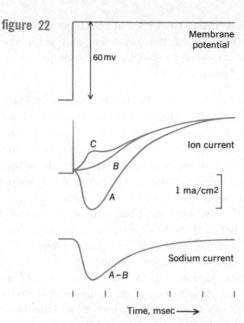

Diagram showing the analysis of ionic membrane current by the voltage-clamp technique. The membrane potential of a squid axon is suddenly displaced from −60 mv to zero (upper trace). The resulting ionic current flow (middle trace; outward current upwards) is recorded under three different conditions: A: axon surrounded by sea water; B: 9/10 of external sodium replaced by choline (approximately equalizing the sodium activities on either side of the membrane); C: external sodium totally replaced by choline. Curve B shows the delayed increase of potassium current by itself. Bottom trace ($A - B$): the difference between curves A and B shows magnitude and time course of the inward directed sodium current when the axon is in sea water. The time course corresponds to an experiment at 8.5°C (after Hodgkin, 1958; Hodgkin and Huxley, 1952b).

tion is lowered, e.g., by replacing NaCl with choline chloride or sucrose, the null point of this component falls in accordance with the Nernst equation: it always follows the equilibrium potential for Na ions.

The conclusion, therefore, is that a suddenly applied and maintained depolarization produces first a rapid increase of Na conductance, this being a transient effect which is converted within a few milliseconds into an increased K conductance (Fig. 23).

It is a matter of special interest that the Na and K permeabilities do not increase simultaneously, but the changes have a different time characteristic and are out of phase. The membrane continues to discriminate between the two ion species even in its depolarized condition, but the ratio of Na/K conductance is temporarily reversed. In the normal course of events, when no provision is made for voltage clamping, the initial change (increase of Na conductance) is a regenerative event leading to the self-reinforcing ascent of the spike. The subsequent process (namely, the cutting off, or "inactivation," of the Na-transfer mechanism and its conversion into a state of greatly increased K conductance) is a self-repairing event. It causes an accelerated efflux of K ions from the axoplasm. This leads to a rapid fall of the inside potential to the initial level, which is automatically followed by a restoration of the original ion permeabilities. Thus, the increase of K conductance

figure 23

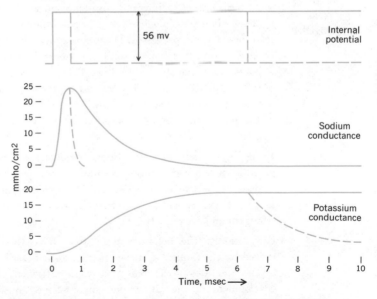

Time course of sodium conductance g_{Na} and potassium conductance g_K associated with a depolarization of 56 mv. (From Hodgkin, 1958.) The continuous curves [which were derived from the results illustrated diagrammatically in Fig. 22, (a) and (b)] are for a maintained voltage step. The broken curves show the effect of repolarizing the membrane after two intervals indicated by broken vertical lines in the trace at the top.

is a process of *negative feedback*, which shuts itself off as it proceeds. It brings about a rapid termination of the active cycle and restoration of the normal excitability of the axon, leaving it in a state of readiness to conduct another impulse within 1 or 2 msec. It may be noted that the existence of a refractory period (p. 24) is the consequence of a transient condition during which the Na gates are shut and the K gates wide open. In this state the membrane potential is driven automatically toward E_K at or even below the resting level (i.e., a more negative level inside) from which it cannot easily be displaced, and the regenerative mechanism is temporarily out of action. However, the refractory state passes off quickly once the membrane potential has returned toward its baseline.

the quantitative reconstruction of the action potential and of its mode of propagation

One of the important results of the voltage-clamp experiments was the accurate measurement of the changes in ionic conductance, or permeability, for various stepwise displacements of the membrane potential. A complete set of measurements with different amounts of depolarization was made, and from these the amplitude and time course of sodium and potassium currents were determined over the whole physiological range of potential levels and analyzed in terms of three processes: (1) increase of sodium permeability, (2) decline (inactivation) of sodium permeability, and (3) increase of potassium permeability (see Figs. 22 to 24). From measurements of the kind illustrated in Figs. 23 and 24, the rate constants of the three processes were calculated and their dependence on the level of the membrane potential was expressed by a set of empirical equations.

Using these quantitative relations, the changes of the membrane potential which occur under normal, "unclamped," conditions in response to electric stimulation could be predicted, and were found to fit the experimental observations with remarkable accuracy (Hodgkin and Huxley, 1952e).

For example, the behavior near and above threshold characterized by the family of curves in Fig. 19 is described accurately by the equations of the ionic theory. In particular, the automatic development of the all-or-none spike above threshold and the underlying cycles of sodium and potassium conductance change are fitted quantitatively by the theory.

The voltage-clamp measurements were made on a long cylindrical piece of axon membrane that was subjected to uniform voltage

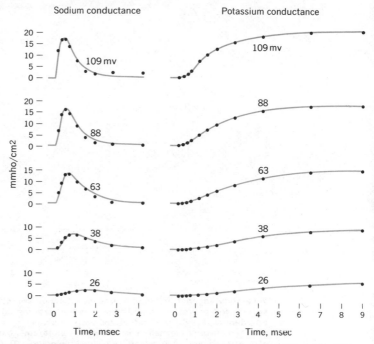

The Increase of sodium and potassium conductances associated with five different displacements of the membrane potential. The depolarization step for each curve is shown by the number, in mv. Time course corresponds to observations at 6°C. (From Hodgkin, 1958.)

control. The results could be used to compute the process of longitudinal propagation of the potential wave along the axon. By "feeding" an electric pulse into a theoretical cable whose properties (internal core resistance, distributed membrane capacity, and voltage-dependent membrane conductances) are identical with those of the axon, the shape of the spike, its all-or-nothing character, the quantities of ion exchange, and the velocity of propagation could be calculated (see Fig. 25). In all these events, the rise of sodium conductance provides the self-reinforcing link, not only in initiating an action potential but in causing activity to spread from point to point at a rate depending on the resistance and capacity of the cable line.

The quick electric restoration of the membrane potential shown in Fig. 25 is not a universal phenomenon; there are several instances, notably the electric response of heart muscle, in which the secondary increase of K permeability does not take place and the

figure 25

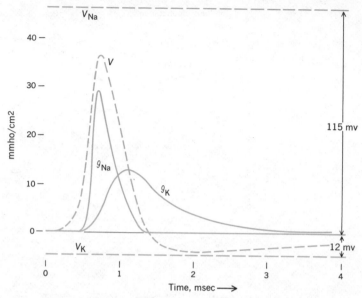

Theoretical reconstruction of a propagated action potential (curve V) and sodium and potassium conductances, using experimental constants appropriate to 18.5°C. Total calculated entry of sodium = 4.33×10^{-12} mole/ cm^2; total loss of potassium = 4.26×10^{-12} mole/cm^2. Calculated velocity of propagation = 18.8 m/sec (observed velocity = 21.2 m/sec). (From Hodgkin and Huxley, 1952e.)

Na conductance does not shut itself off completely. The result is the appearance of a prolonged plateau of depolarization in the heart action potential whose functional significance is that it provides a sufficiently long-maintained stimulus for the systolic contraction of the heart muscle fibers.

After an action-potential wave has passed and the initial levels of potential, ionic conductance, and excitability have been restored, the residual change is a minute deficit of the intracellular potassium store. Sodium has entered the cytoplasm and potassium has been lost in the amount of approximately 3 to 4×10^{-12} mole/cm^2 of cell surface (p. 81). In terms of ion concentration, the internal potassium level of a squid axon has declined by about 1/1,000,000. This is a very small loss, which would be repaid in a few seconds by the Na/K pump working at a slightly accelerated rate. It is not surprising that even if the pump has been stopped by metabolic inhibitors, a squid axon is capable of producing a few hundred thousand impulses simply by drawing on its accumulated ion store without recharging it (Hodgkin, 1964). In most excitable cells, intense activity is an intermittent (in some nerve cells, diurnal) phenomenon, and chemical recovery processes are used to build up and maintain a long-term reservoir of free energy rather than to replenish losses immediately or "top up" ionic concentrations during each interval between impulses. This principle of "brief bursts of high-rate activity, followed by long periods of chemical restoration," applies to skeletal muscle and to most of our nerve cells, with the obvious exception of rythmically active tissues, e.g., the heart and respiratory muscles and the nerve cells concerned with them.

The quantity of charge transferred during an impulse across 1 cm^2 of membrane is approximately the same in different nonmyelinated nerve fibers. This is a consequence of the approximate constancy of the membrane capacity (1 $\mu f/cm^2$) and of the constant amplitude of resting and action potentials in different cells. It follows that the intracellular concentration change and the percentage loss of potassium will be about 1,000 times larger in a very small axon, say of 0.5-μ diameter, than in the giant axon of the squid. Thus the signaling capacity of a nerve fiber depends to some extent on its size: the smaller the fiber, the greater its dependence on a continuous metabolic supply of energy to extrude Na and regain K ions, which have exchanged during "busy" periods of signaling activity.

There are several physical and chemical signs which accompany the long recovery process after intense nerve activity: the fibers produce extra heat and consume oxygen above the normal resting rate; this is associated with accelerated extrusion of Na and accumulation of K by the axon, and at the same time a small increase in membrane potential ("hyperpolarization") is often observed (cf. p. 66).

In addition to the prolonged recovery heat production, an early transient phase of thermal exchange has been discovered by A. V. Hill and his coworkers (see Hill, 1932), who used extremely sensitive recording methods. This phase is of special interest because it either accompanies or very rapidly follows the passage of an impulse. This phenomenon of "initial nerve heat" is indicative of a chemical reaction occurring immediately after, or even during, the permeability change itself. The total amount of heat liberated during this early phase is minute, and Hill has suggested that if there is a process of membrane reorganization that in any way resembles a chemical breakdown, it can involve only a few scattered molecular sites. The same general conclusion has been reached by a very different, electrical, approach. Cole and Curtis (1939) found a drastic "resistance breakdown" of the axon membrane during excitation: the resistance of 1 cm^2 of membrane fell from 1,000 to approximately 20 ohms, and the capacity remained at 1 $\mu f/cm^2$. But for a surface layer of 50 Å thickness, this result means that its specific resistance is still 10^6 times higher than that of the surrounding medium (instead of nearly 10^8 times; see p. 48). The "bulk" of the membrane material retains its dielectric properties and continues to behave like an insulating condenser of fixed capacity. The ionic conductance change presumably occurs at small scattered sites that take up altogether less than 1% of the axon surface. The momentary leakage of Na and K during the impulse (3 to 4×10^{-12} mole/cm^2) results in an *average* transfer of one ion at points about 70 Å apart. If this process is mediated by activation of special "carrier molecules," each of which transports a large number of ions, the ionic flux would be concentrated at far fewer sites much further apart.

One of the few outstanding remaining problems concerns the physicochemical nature of the permeability change and the mechanism of its electrical control.

It has been claimed that a local release and turnover of acetylcholine is responsible for membrane excitation and for its underlying permeability change (Nachmansohn, 1959). But although this view has aroused much interest, it has not so far been based on adequate experimental evidence (see discussions by del Castillo and Katz, 1956, and Katz, 1960).*

* Nachmansohn's view was developed from the observation that doses of anticholinesterases that are sufficient to inhibit the intracellular hydrolysis of acetylcholine will block impulses in nerve and muscle. Criticism has been directed against the far-reaching nature of Nachmansohn's arguments, which, to the minds of many investigators, are not acceptable without more direct evidence. The basic factual claims underlying Nachmansohn's hypothesis have meanwhile also been rendered untenable by the well-designed and carefully controlled experiments of Feng and Hsieh (1952a and 1952b). With the use of an irreversible cholinesterase inhibitor (tetraethyl pyrophosphate), Feng and Hsieh showed that the enzyme activity of frog nerves and muscles can be eliminated without reducing the size of the action potential.

6
the propagation
of the impulse

The effect of the regenerative entry of sodium is to produce an all-or-none response once the threshold potential (i.e., the unstable "ignition point" of the system) has been exceeded. In this way, the axon membrane can amplify a threshold change of, say, 20 mv by a factor of 5, thus automatically compensating for the defects of its cable structure. The large potential change propagates along the whole length of the axon without decreasing in amplitude. If one applies a "local anesthetic" like procaine to a region of the axon, this abolishes the regenerative entry of sodium without greatly altering the passive cable properties of the fiber. It has been found that a minimum length of the fiber must be paralyzed before an impulse is actually blocked. This is because the action potential arriving at the inexcitable region is a powerful electric stimulus that has a large margin of safety (about 5:1). Although it would be attenuated by passive cable spread, it would still have enough signal strength left at the other end of a short, say 1 mm, inexcitable length of fiber to reexcite the membrane and so carry on the rest of the way.

When compared with the transmission of messages in an efficient cable, the triggered all-or-none character of the nerve impulse has an obvious and important drawback. It reduces the signal-carrying capacity of an axon to a fixed wave form that is capable of very little variation in either amplitude or shape. The nerve impulse is, in fact, merely a stereotype code element, like the "dot" of the Morse code. This means that in a brief time interval not very much information can be transmitted in any one single fiber, and a large multiplicity of parallel lines must be provided wherever detailed information is to be conveyed, e.g., in the channel between eye and brain.

At the different sensory nerve endings, specific stimuli depolarize the axon terminals and so initiate a sequence of all-or-none impulses in the individual fibers (see Adrian, 1928, 1932, 1947; Matthews, 1931; Katz, 1950; Eyzaguirre and Kuffler, 1955; Granit, 1955; Bullock, 1959; Gray, 1959; Hartline, 1959; Schmitt, 1959).

The velocity of the impulse depends on the rate at which the membrane capacity ahead of the impulse is discharged beyond the threshold level. This in turn depends on both the cable constants of the fiber (principally its surface capacity and the longitudinal resistances of the fiber core and the external medium) and on the "safety margin" of the impulse (i.e., how much current it can generate in excess of the threshold requirement of the resting fiber). Because the velocity of the wave depends on the longitudinal conductance of the axon core, it is closely related to the fiber size. *Theoretically*, in nonmyelinated axons and muscle fibers, one would expect the propagation velocity to increase with the square root of the diameter, other factors being equal (Rushton, 1951, and Hodgkin, 1954).* Empirically this relation does not always fit, and some authors favor a linear relationship. In any case, it is agreed that one way of obtaining a higher speed of signal transmission is to lower the axial cable resistance by increasing the fiber size. This is a solution chosen by Nature for certain high-speed requirements of invertebrate animals. For example, the rapid escape

---

* The phrase "other factors being equal" means that in comparing fibers of different size their specific electric properties are assumed to remain the same (e.g., time constants, *specific* capacitance and resistances of membrane and cytoplasm, and current density per unit area of membrane). The following relations can then be applied.

1. Longitudinal current along the axon core is

$$i_{long} = -\frac{1}{r_i}\frac{dv}{dx} \quad [\text{cf. Eq. (7)}]$$

where r_i = core resistance per cm length of axon

v = internal potential

Now,

$$r_i = \frac{4R_i}{\pi D^2}$$

where D = fiber diameter

R_i = specific resistance of the axoplasm, taken to be the same among comparable fibers of different diameters.

If the axon is immersed in a large volume of solution, the outside resistance is negligible and external potential can be ignored.

2. The membrane current per unit length is

movement of the squid is controlled by the few giant axons supplying its large "jet propelling" mantle muscle. The development of giant axons would not be a practical proposition for an animal that needs not only speed but a great multiplicity of signal channels in order to achieve fine gradation of its sensory or motor traffic. It is clear, for instance, that there would be no room for many giant fibers in our optic nerve, where more than 1 million axons are needed side-by-side to convey visual information at high speed.

The solution that was provided in the vertebrate nervous system was the development of the medullated axon, in which cable losses are greatly reduced by the use of the myelin sheath.

In the nonmyelinated fiber (axon or muscle fiber), the membrane is either relatively freely exposed to the external conducting medium (muscle) or invested with a very thin layer of satellite (Schwann) cells, whose interstices provide numerous low-resistance pathways between the lymphatic fluid and the axon surface. The regenerative process of excitation presumably occurs at numerous sites scattered all along the membrane, either in random distribution or spatially linked to the frequent gaps in the Schwann cell cover.

The medullated axon, on the other hand, is provided with a segmented insulating sleeve of low capacity. According to electron-

$$i_m = -\frac{di_{long}}{dx} = \frac{1}{r_i}\frac{d^2v}{dx^2} = \frac{\pi D^0}{4 R_i}\frac{d^2v}{dx^2}$$

The density of the membrane current per unit surface area is

$$I_m = \frac{D}{4R_i}\frac{d^2v}{dx^2}$$

For a potential wave traveling at constant velocity θ,

$$\frac{dv}{dx} = \frac{1}{\theta}\frac{dv}{dt}$$

and

$$\frac{d^2v}{dx^2} = \frac{1}{\theta^2}\frac{d^2v}{dt^2}$$

Hence

$$I_m = \frac{D}{4R_i\theta^2}\frac{d^2v}{dt^2}$$

If the specific membrane properties remain the same for fibers of different size, the time course of the potential wave passing any one point and the current density through the membrane during the passage of the wave also remain the same (while the wave length changes with the velocity). It follows that D/θ^2 is constant, and conduction velocity θ varies with the square root of the fiber diameter.

microscope evidence each segment is formed by multiple spiral wrappings of a Schwann cell winding itself tightly around the axon cylinder. The whole system forms a much better analogy to a miniature submarine cable than does the nonmyelinated fiber. There is ordinary passive cable transmission of the spike potential along each myelin-covered segment. Along this distance of 1 to 2 mm, some attenuation of the signal occurs, but the losses are not severe, and the active relay mechanism is restricted to discrete sites, namely, the small exposed membrane surface at each node of Ranvier (Tasaki, 1939, 1953; Huxley and Stämpfli, 1949; Frankenhaeuser, 1952, 1960). This provides a signaling channel of much higher speed and metabolic economy than a nonmedullated axon of the same size, and it enables us to carry a much greater number of separate high-speed communication channels packed into a small bundle.

generality of the ionic theory The most detailed and cogent evidence for the important role of sodium and potassium ions in the conduction of the nerve signal has been obtained on a particularly favorable, but also rather unusual, preparation—the giant nerve fibers of the squid. Parallel experiments of an inevitably less stringent kind have been made on many other excitable tissues, and certain limits to the generalization of the Na/K theory have indeed been discovered. The role of sodium in the process of electric excitation appears to be very similar in vertebrate skeletal muscle ("twitch type"), myelinated and nonmyelinated axons, and heart muscle.

The generalization does not seem to apply to the action potentials that can be recorded in crustacean muscle and certain conducting plant cells. In these tissues, the situation has not yet been fully explored. In its kinetic behavior, the process of excitation seems to be completely analogous to that illustrated in Fig. 19 above, but the nature of the principal ionic channels is not the same. Instead of Na entry, efflux of an internal anion (Cl⁻ in the case of Nitella; see Gaffey and Mullins, 1958) and entry of a divalent cation like Ca (Fatt and Ginsborg, 1958) have been cited as regenerative factors.

In most of the conducting nerve and muscle cells so far studied, sodium is the only normally occurring ion that can supply the regenerative inward current during excitation, but in all cases some foreign cations have been found that can be used effectively as a sodium substitute. The best known is lithium, whose ability to replace sodium in electric excitation of muscle was first demonstrated by Overton (1902). In some cells, various quaternary ammonium ions and related compounds can restore the regenerative process after it has been suspended by withdrawal of sodium, but it is not yet clear whether these organic ions simply take over the place of sodium and move through its normal membrane channels or whether they act by modifying the properties of the membrane in such a way that other ions, e.g., calcium, can produce or effectively contribute to the regenerative flow of inward current.

conduction
with
decrement

In the normal axon or skeletal muscle fiber, there is a sharp *ignition point*—the threshold potential at which the impulse arises explosively in an all-or-none manner and then propagates without attenuation, or decrement. Yet, we know that the underlying mechanism is a continuously graded process that is dependent on a nonlinear relation between membrane voltage and ion permeability. This is evident even below threshold, as was recognized for many years, in the voltage/current characteristic of the membrane and the associated local response. The added contribution which the regenerative but still subthreshold sodium entry makes to the induced depolarization shows up as an increment in the voltage/current slope, and in several respects this simulates a local increase of the membrane resistance. Thus the appearance of a local response is associated with an increased spatial spread of the potential change away from its origin, the change being still decremental but with a greater effective "length constant" than one observes with smaller or with opposite potential changes.

In certain tissues, and in all tissues under certain abnormal conditions, the regenerating process is too weak to support a propagating spike without energy being supplied by an external stimulating source (or by a synaptic transmitter action). This happens in many arthropod muscles, and possibly also in the cell body and dendrites of some neurons. It is a state which can be compared with that of a partially refractory axon membrane with the *sodium* mechanism largely inactivated and the *potassium* mechanism operating at full efficiency. In this state, there is no critical threshold and no all-or-none response. One obtains action potentials which have rates of rise and peak amplitudes that depend upon the strength of the initiating stimulus and which progressively decline and fade out within several millimeters of fiber length. They are, in fact, an exaggerated form of local response and are distinguished from the conventional local action potential only by the fact that they continue to rise after the end of an applied brief current pulse for a short period that is terminated by accelerated potassium efflux (or an analogous process of electric restoration). Lorente de Nó and Condouris (1959) have suggested that such attenuated action potentials may have considerable functional importance; for instance, if the dendrites of central nerve cells behave in this manner, decremental spikes would make a significant contribution to the integration of excitatory events at converging synapses by reinforcing the ordinary local spread of subthreshold potentials within the postsynaptic neuron.

7

transmission of impulses within cells and across cell boundaries

In the preceding chapter, we discussed the mechanism by which messages are propagated within the boundaries of single cells. This is essentially a two-stage process and is dependent on (1) the cable properties of the cell, which, though imperfect, enable electrical signals to spread forward over a short distance, and (2) an electrochemical relay mechanism built into the cell membrane, which automatically boosts the signal to full strength all along the line and so makes up for the imperfections of the cable structure.

What happens at a synapse (p. 3) when an impulse reaches the terminal end of a nerve fiber? According to the neuron theory (p. 5), the synapse is a functional contact between two excitable cells whose cytoplasms are enclosed within separate membranes. This view has received firm support from observations with the electron microscope which have shown not only the presence of separate membranes but of a space between the presynaptic and postsynaptic cells amounting to about 150 to 200 Å in many instances.

At the vertebrate neuromuscular junction, the intercellular space is even wider and forms a "gap" of 500 to 1,000 Å. This is partitioned by a fibrous layer (basement membrane) which can be traced all around the surface of the muscle fiber. A structural arrangement of this kind seems incompatible with a continuation of the electric cable process across the junction. If one assumes the electric resistances and capacities of the synaptic membranes and intercellular spaces to be about the same as those known to exist along the rest of the fibers, the action current produced by the motor nerve endings could not depolarize the muscle membrane by more than a fraction of a microvolt (p. 113).

Such calculations, however, are beset with uncertainty, for the electron microscope tells us nothing about the electrical properties of membrane and interspaces and these may well be different at synaptic junctions from what has been measured elsewhere. Moreover, there is a great deal of structural variation between different synapses. In some, the cell membranes show regions of much closer proximity, and in certain types of junctions, actual fusion of presynaptic and postsynaptic membranes has been described (Hama, 1961, 1962, and Bennett et al., 1963). Such features are of great interest; they appear to be related to the two different modes of transmission, chemical and electric, which occur at different types of synapses (see Katz, 1958). There is increasing evidence suggesting that membrane fusion (the so-called "tight junction") may be a structural basis for electric coupling between two cells.

Some of the most interesting structures revealed by the electron microscope are the so-called presynaptic vesicles. They have been found densely accumulated inside many nerve terminals in the peripheral as well as central nervous system. Masses of vesicles, of about 500-Å diameter, are concentrated near the synaptic contact points of those nerve endings whose function depends on the release of a specific transmitter substance.

The discovery of presynaptic vesicles coincided with the physiological finding that the transmitter substance acetylcholine is secreted from motor nerve terminals in minimum packets of large, multimolecular size. It has been suggested that the vesicles are the structural units responsible for this "quantal release" (del Castillo and Katz, 1955, and Palay, 1956).*

---

* This hypothesis was based originally on experimental results obtained at the neuromuscular junction, and has since been extended to many other types of "chemically operating" synapses. The justification must depend, in each case, on evidence for a quantal mechanism of transmitter release and for a terminal localization of presynaptic vesicles. Attempts have been made to go further and, by generalization, to classify all neuronal structures which contain vesicles as "chemically transmitting presynaptic terminals." Without more direct evidence, this would be difficult to defend because the presence of vesicles, though characteristic of such terminals, is certainly not restricted to them. It would indeed be most surprising if simple subcellular particles like vesicles, which can be found in endothelial cells as well as nerve cells, did not serve a variety of very different functions in their different situations.

electrical and chemical transmission at synapses

The dispute between *continuity* and *contact* theories had a curious parallel in the physiological field. The functional continuity concept was represented by the theory that the transmission of impulses across synapses is essentially a continuation of the process by which impulses are conducted within the boundaries of each individual cell. Opposed to this was the view that in synaptic transmission the intervention of chemical mediators is required and that the unicellular mechanism of propagation by electric currents comes to a stop at the presynaptic endings, where special transmitter substances are released, after which they take control of the synaptic process. The presence of closed terminal membranes and extracellular spaces between two cells could not fail to impede the propagation of the nerve message by the ordinary electric process if the membranes have the same insulating qualities and the material of the external spaces has the same conducting properties at the synapses as elsewhere.

In spite of the uncertainties attached to this argument, it is of interest to consider some of its implications quantitatively. We know the order of magnitude of the cable constants, the leakage resistance and capacity of the axon membrane, and the conductivity of the cytoplasmic core. They are of the order of $R_m = 2000$ ohm-cm^2, $C_m = 1$ μf/cm^2, and $R_i = 200$ ohm-cm.* When a nerve impulse travels along a nonmyelinated fiber of, say, 5-μ diameter, it faces at every point a leaky cable with an input impedance of approximately 20 megohms.† To activate the membrane just ahead of the impulse, sufficient current must flow into it to lower the existing resting potential across the membrane by about 20 mv. When this level is reached, excitation occurs, and as a result of excitation the potential change, brought about by the cable currents from the advancing wave of activity, is amplified about

---

* R_m is the specific transverse resistance of a unit area (1 cm^2) of membrane, C_m is the specific capacity of a unit area of membrane, and R_i is the specific resistance across a 1-cm cube of cytoplasm. (Note that membrane resistance decreases, while capacity increases, with increasing surface area; hence the dimensions of ohm $\times$ cm^2 and μf/cm^2.)

† The input impedance Z is derived from the following equation

$$Z = \sqrt{R_m R_i/(2\pi^2\rho^3 \sqrt{1 + 4\pi^2 f^2 R_m^2 C_m^2})}$$

where ρ is fiber radius and f the alternating current frequency at which Z is determined (with action potentials of the usual time course, 250 cycles/sec is an approximate value for f).

five to ten times and so produces sufficient current to excite the region ahead in a similar fashion.

Any physical or chemical agent that interferes with this automatic process of amplification (e.g., local cooling, pressure, application of procaine) will act as a local "anesthetic" and block the propagation of the impulse (Hodgkin, 1937). Because of the large normal safety margin, it is generally not sufficient to render the axon inexcitable at a "point," or at a single node of Ranvier. So long as the cable properties of the fiber remain intact, the passive electric spread of potential will enable it to "jump" across a short inexcitable region. Provided the signal is not attenuated to less than $\frac{1}{5}$, the threshold level will be attained on the other side of the "block" and propagation will then be resumed. To produce an impassable blockage, a sufficient length of fiber must be anesthetized—generally one or a few millimeters—to cause the voltage of the signal, spreading by cable action to the other side beyond the block, to become attenuated to less than threshold (see Hodgkin, 1937; reviewed by Katz, 1939).

An alternative way of blocking impulse propagation would be to interfere locally with the electric continuity of the cable structure. Suppose one closes the core of the $5\text{-}\mu$ axon by placing a membrane

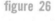

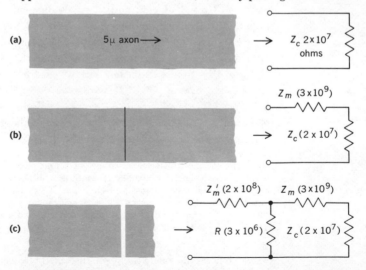

Input impedance for the impulse during axonal conduction (a) and at "model synapse" (b and c). Z_c = input impedance of axon. Z_m, Z_m' = terminal membrane impedance (resting and activated, respectively).

septum across it, as in diagram (*b*) of Fig. 26. If this septum had the same specific resistance as the surface membrane, it would amount to placing no less than 3,000 megohms across the line in front of the cable impedance of 20 megohms. The efficacy of the action current would therefore be reduced by the septum to less than 1% and conduction would undoubtedly fail.

Now suppose one divides the axon in two, closes each end with a membrane of the usual electric properties, and separates the terminal ends by a gap 150Å wide. We then get the type of cell contact, or synapse, that has been described for various tissues. The situation is now far worse than it was in the case of a single septum. It is easy to show that if the physical properties of the synaptic structures are similar to those of the rest of the cell, electric transmission will be completely ineffective, except perhaps in the case of very large "giant" fibers.

The situation we have now is that instead of a continuous cable, there are two cable structures that are connected electrically by an attenuating network of very high losses. The network is made up by the series impedance of the terminal prefiber membrane, the shunt resistance of the 150-Å gap, and another series impedance due to the terminal postfiber membrane.* Let us suppose the prefiber membrane becomes activated and its resistance falls from 2,000 to 40 ohm-cm^2. Even then, the electric attenuation of a brief voltage signal like the impulse across this synapse amounts to $(3 \times 10^6)/(2 \times 10^8) \times (2 \times 10^7)/(3 \times 10^9) = 10^{-4}$. There are many synapses where the possibility of continuous electric transmission seems even more remote. To these belong the nerve-muscle junctions of vertebrate animals, in which the gap between the contacting cells is greater and the muscle fiber, being of much larger diameter, has a much lower input impedance and a much greater demand for current supply than its supplying axon branches.

But there are also some junctions where the situation, from an electric point of view, is more favorable than in the 5-μ fibers, which we have so far considered. The interesting point is that the shunt resistance R of our 150-Å gap stays constant at about 3

---

* The terms "prefiber" and "postfiber" denote in short the presynaptic and postsynaptic cells, respectively.

megohms independent of the diameter of the contacting cells ($R = \zeta/8\pi d$) where ζ is the specific resistance of the gap material and d the width of the gap. On the other hand, the terminal membrane impedance falls with the inverse square of the fiber size. Hence, for the segmental synapses in the giant fiber system of a worm or arthropod, the attenuation across the septa would be 1/10 instead of 1/10,000, which brings us close to the range in which electric transmission becomes possible. All one needs is a moderate further lowering of the terminal membrane impedance, and the observed continuity of transmission in both directions is achieved.

Returning to the small, 5-μ junction, we concluded that electric transmission across a 150-Å gap was out of the question. However, our calculations were based on the assumption that the electrical properties of the terminal membranes and of the extracellular gap material were much the same as elsewhere. This may be wrong, and it is worth inquiring how far one would have to reduce the terminal insulation resistance to ensure the forward travel of the signal by electrical means. The answer is, from the usual 2,000 ohms $\times$ cm² to less than 1 ohm $\times$ cm², which is less than one generally encounters among axon membranes but is not impossible.

An alternative way of overcoming the impasse at this junction would be to establish minute cytoplasmic bridges. Suppose we allowed our synapses to be crossed by minute bridges about 100 Å thick. How many such bridges are necessary to enable the cable current from our prefiber to excite the postfiber? The answer is about 20, or one bridge per square micron, which occupies less than 1/10,000 of the cross-sectional area of the gap. No such bridges have been seen in the electron microscope, but it remains possible that scattered, small connections of this kind may exist in the case of special junctions (for instance at the cell contacts between heart muscle fibers), although they are technically difficult to detect.

There is good evidence that synaptic gaps are not without some structural detail (de Robertis, 1962, 1964). There are even cases, exemplified by the work on tissue fragments of Gray and Whittaker (1962), and de Robertis et al. (1961), in which the postsynaptic membrane was found to be more firmly attached to the presynaptic endings than to the remainder of its own cell wall. How-

ever, the fine details of such connections have not yet been resolved. It will be an important task to clear up the nature of the
structural links between synaptically contacting cells and to make
certain that scattered protoplasmic bridges of small diameter
have not been overlooked.

So far, we have considered—in a speculative manner—two ways by
which Nature might establish continuity of electric transmission
between two cells in spite of their apparent structural separation.
There are several known cases of cellular contacts which behave
like an electrical "syncytium" (in certain smooth muscles, in heart
muscle, and in the segmental septa of invertebrate giant nerve
fibers). In these cases, adjoining cells form electrical cable connections of sufficiently low internal core resistance, and impulses are
conducted with apparently equal ease in either direction. The only
structural modifications which have been described at some of
these electrical synapses and which may be relevant are certain
regions where the intercellular gap is greatly reduced and where
even fusion of the two membranes occurs. To enable the cells to
function as electrical units, such membrane regions must have
very low resistance; i.e., they either have many holes of molecular
size—which is the first possibility mentioned on p. 102—or few
holes of large size—the second proposition considered above. It is
to be hoped that further advances with the electron microscope
will allow one to decide between these possibilities.

To apply the word "synapse" to the cell connections in the heart
or in the giant fibers of invertebrate nerve cords is really a mis-
nomer. The functional behavior of these tissues is that of a
syncytial unit in which excitation spreads from one point to the
next in much the same way as within a single cell. By contrast, the
term "synapse" is customarily reserved for those cell connections
which allow an excitation wave, (or, more generally, an excitatory
or inhibitory influence) to pass in only one, but not in the reverse,
direction.* Synapses are the "one-way valves" of our signal traffic;
it is this property of the synaptic connection that ensures that
nerve fibers are used almost exclusively for one-way traffic in

---

* An interesting exception has been brought to light by Martin and Pilar
(1963a and 1963b), who found that the synapses in the ciliary ganglion
of the chick provide a sufficiently close "electric coupling" for action
currents to spread effectively in both orthodromic and antidromic
directions.

normal life (even though they are quite capable of conducting an impulse with equal facility in both directions).

Even if we restrict our attention to one-way synapses, it is not possible to make a general statement about their mode of operation. It has been found by experiment that at different synapses, different kinds of mechanisms are at work, the main division being between electrical and chemical types of transmission.

electrical transmission at excitatory and inhibitory synapses

Convincing evidence for an electrical mechanism has been obtained by Furshpan and Potter (1959) for an excitatory synapse in the crayfish abdominal nerve cord and by Furukawa and Furshpan (1963) for an inhibitory connection made with the large Mauthner cell of the goldfish brain.

The abdominal cord of the crayfish contains large synaptic contacts between a "giant fiber," which runs along the cord on each side, and the segmental motor axons, which supply the rapid flexor muscle of the "tail." Impulses are transmitted across this connection from the giant fiber to the motor axon, but not in the opposite direction. The fine structure of the synapse shows little bulbous processes of the motor axon, which fit closely into presynaptic "sockets," i.e., small cavities in the surface of the giant axon. According to de Lorenzo (1959), Hama (1961), and Robertson (1961), the membranes in this "ball-and-socket" joint approach one another closely and in some places seem to be fused together.

Furshpan and Potter studied the electric conductivity of this synapse by inserting electrodes on each side of the junction so as to pass current and measure voltage changes across the presynaptic and postsynaptic membrane. They found that the synaptic contact acts as a good electric rectifying element and allows current to pass along the core in the forward direction, that is, from the presynaptic to the postsynaptic axoplasm, but not in the reverse direction. The result was that, experimentally, subthreshold electric "signals" could be transferred from one cell to the other, provided the internal potential of the prefiber was made higher (more positive) than that of the postfiber. This can be achieved either by locally depolarizing the presynaptic axon (i.e., making its inside *less* negative) or hyperpolarizing the postsynaptic axon (making its interior *more* negative). In other words, this neuronal junction is capable of transmitting *depolarization* (and therefore also the action potential) in the *normal* direction and *hyperpolarization* (produced by applied current) in the *antidromic* direction.

This was an interesting discovery. That nerve and muscle membranes can act effectively as electric rectifiers had been known for many years, but this was the first instance in which the rectifying property of a membrane contact was found to ensure one-way transmission of impulses across a synaptic junction.

The more one finds out about properties of different synapses, the less grows one's inclination to make general statements about their mode of action! In the squid stellate ganglion, there are the "giant synapses" between the endings of a large central axon and the giant motor axon which supplies the jet-propelling mantle muscle—a situation which resembles superficially that in the crayfish cord. Yet, Hagiwara and Tasaki (1958), who carried out a series of experiments rather similar to those of Furshpan and Potter, could find no evidence for direct electric transmission in the squid synapse, and their results strongly suggest that there is no measurable "cable transmission" in either direction across this cell junction. It is of interest, incidentally, that in the electron microscope (Hama, 1962), this synapse differs from the one in the crayfish and resembles the more conventional type in that it possesses characteristic clusters of vesicles piled up against the presynaptic membrane and, apparently, complete separation of the cell membranes without regions of local fusion.

In a more recent paper, Furukawa and Furshpan (1963) investigated a synapse on the Mauthner neuron of the goldfish, at which *inhibition* is produced electrically by the action currents of the presynaptic fibers. It was known that, under certain conditions, the action currents of a nerve fiber can "inhibit," i.e., reduce the excitability of, a neighboring fiber (Katz and Schmitt, 1940, and Marrazzi and Lorente de Nó, 1944). To see this effect, one must raise the electric resistance around the fibers so that the action currents produce large potential changes on the outside of the axon and an appreciable fraction of the current penetrates the adjacent resting cell. Such conditions are obtained when one places an isolated bundle of axons into an electrically insulating medium, but the effect is absent or very small *in situ*, where the cells are surrounded by a large amount of conducting tissue spaces. Fursh-pan and Furukawa (1962) showed that the so-called "axon cap" of the Mauthner cell is a specialized region in which the extra-cellular resistance is high (possibly because of a dense packing of nerve or glia cells). If one places an electrode into this region, one records very large external action potentials from the adjacent nerve cells. When a volley of impulses approaches the Mauthner cell in the closely packed presynaptic nerve branches, the action currents that emerge from them raise the potential on the outside of the Mauthner cell by many (up to 18) millivolts. A substantial current enters the postsynaptic membrane in this region (leaving the cell at more distant, nonsynaptic, points). This hyperpolarizes the cell in the region in which it is most excitable and in which impulses normally arise and so produces effective inhibition. Furukawa and Furshpan point out that at the same or closely adjacent synapses of the Mauthner cell, another—very different—inhibitory process is at work, which involves the release of a trans-mitter substance and leads to a slower and more lasting effect on the postsynaptic membrane.

examples of chemical transmission at synapses

The first convincing demonstration of chemical transmission was obtained by Otto Loewi in 1921. Impulses in the vagus nerve inhibit the contraction of the heart muscle (amplitude and fre-quency of the beat are reduced). Loewi showed that stimulation of the cardiac branch of the vagus causes an inhibitory substance to appear in the fluid of a frog's heart. By the simple process of transferring the fluid sample with a pipette, one can produce sim-ilar inhibition in a second heart. Loewi called this substance the "Vagusstoff" and subsequently identified it as acetylcholine (Table 4). Loewi and his colleagues showed that this substance is released in minute amounts. It is extremely potent, but is also rapidly hydrolyzed by a specific enzyme (or group of enzymes), cholinesterase. The esterase activity can be blocked by a number of specific inhibitors, and Loewi and Navratil (1926) were the first to show that a well-known drug, eserine or physostigmine (see Table 4), owes its powerful pharmacological action to its anti-cholinesterase effect; i.e., it causes the transient synaptic effects of acetylcholine, which is released in the normal course of activity from millions of different nerve endings, to become excessively prolonged and intensified.

The heart muscle is innervated by two mutually antagonistic kinds of nerve: the parasympathetic vagus nerve, which slows the beat, and the sympathetic fibers, which accelerate it. Loewi showed that impulses in the sympathetic fibers act also by releasing a chemical transmitter whose effects can be transferred to another heart. He called this the "accelerating substance"; others referred to it as "sympathin." Many years earlier, Elliott (1904) had pointed out a close similarity between the action of adrenaline and that of sympathetic nerve stimulation, and it seemed fairly clear that the accelerating transmitter was adrenaline or a chemically related substance [later identified as noradrenaline by von Euler (1946)].

Otto Loewi's discovery was the beginning of a line of experimentation that is still being pursued today, that is, the study of chemical transmission at synapses. This includes such diverse problems as the search for different transmitter substances and the attempt to identify them, the inquiry into pathways of intracellular synthesis of such substances, the mechanism by which the impulse releases them (a special case of what is called neurosecretion), and, finally, the mechanism of their postsynaptic action (the combination with specific receptor molecules and the production of physicochemical changes in the cell membrane leading to excitation or inhibition).

Loewi's original experiment was striking in its simplicity; it also showed up one of the limitations of this experimental approach. The transmitter substance is released by nerve impulses in such minute amounts that it can be detected and identified only by biological assay—a method that has obvious disadvantages when compared with direct chemical identification. The frog's heart was a particularly fortunate object of study, for its sensitivity is very high and the transmitter substances are released in sufficient amounts to be assayed directly on a second identical preparation. This could not be achieved in most of the other cases which have since been examined; the amounts of acetylcholine that are released by motor nerves or by the presynaptic fibers in a sympathetic ganglion are so small and become so diluted in the perfusion fluid that they cannot be tested on the same kind of tissue; much more sensitive objects (such as the body wall of the leech, the frog's rectus abdominis muscle, or the heart) must be chosen to assay them.

table 4 Chemical transmitters (acetylcholine, noradrenaline) and other substances of "synaptic potency"

(a) Acetylcholine-like agents

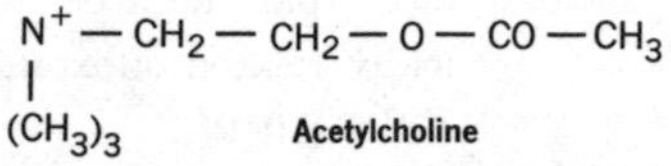

$$N^+ - CH_2 - CH_2 - O - CO - CH_3$$
$$|$$
$$(CH_3)_3 \quad \textbf{Acetylcholine}$$

$$N^+ - CH_2 - CH_2 - O - CO - NH_2$$
$$|$$
$$(CH_3)_3 \quad \textbf{Carbachol}$$

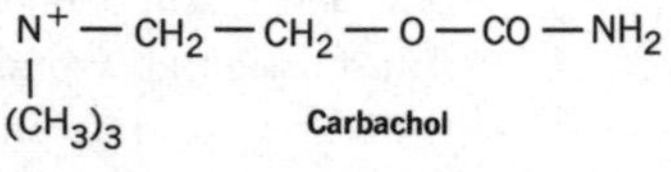

Succinylcholine

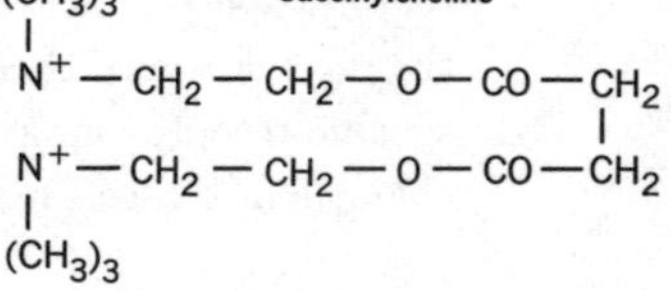

$$(CH_3)_3$$
$$|$$
$$N^+ - CH_2 - CH_2 - O - CO - CH_2$$
$$|$$
$$N^+ - CH_2 - CH_2 - O - CO - CH_2$$
$$|$$
$$(CH_3)_3$$

(b) Adrenergic system

Adrenaline

$(-CH_3) \longrightarrow$

Noradrenaline

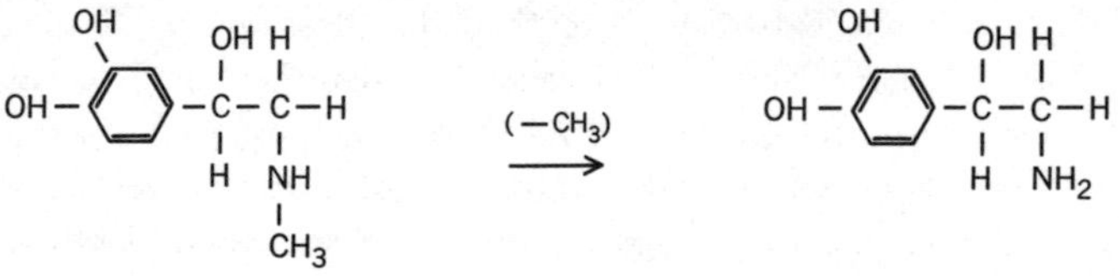

Acetylcholine-blocking agents

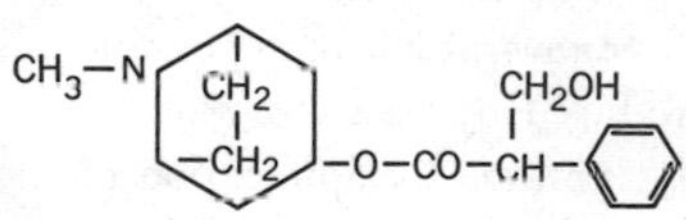

**Anticholinesterases
(Acetylcholine-potentiating agents)**

d-Tubocurarine

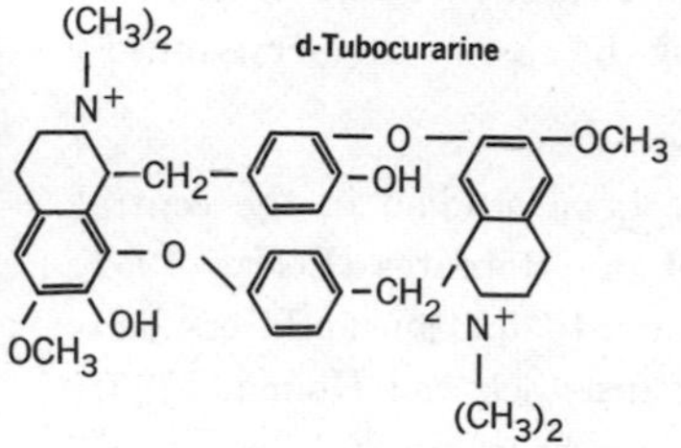

$(CH_3)_2$

Eserine

$CH_3-NH-CO-O-$

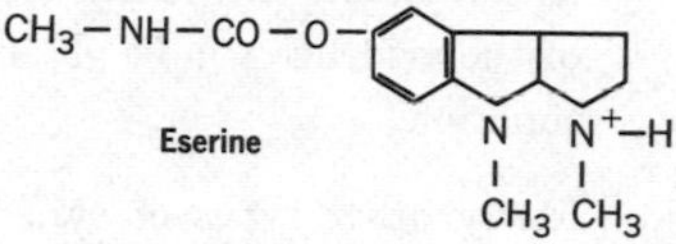

Neostigmine

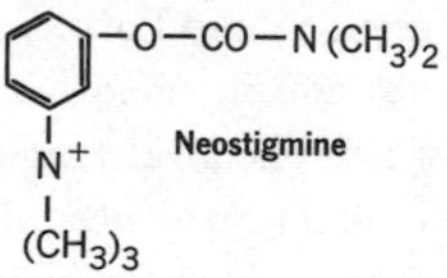

$-O-CO-N(CH_3)_2$

$(CH_3)_3$

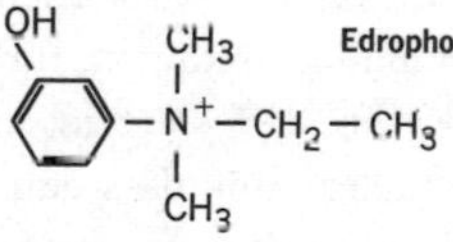

Atropine

Edrophonium

CH_3-N

CH_2OH

Glutamic acid

COOH
|
CH_2
|
CH_2
|
$CHNH_2$
|
COOH

$(-CO_2)$
$\longrightarrow$

$\gamma-$ amino butyric acid

COOH
|
CH_2
|
CH_2
|
CH_2NH_2

(c)   Amino acid system

The present state of the evidence for chemical transmission at synapses can be summarized as follows. The evidence is very strong in the case of the vertebrate nerve-muscle system and the vertebrate autonomic nervous system. In these situations, the release of transmitters has been revealed by assaying the perfusion fluid collected during periods of presynaptic stimulation, and the substances have been identified (as far as a multiple pharmacological-assay technique enables one to do so) as acetylcholine in the nerve-muscle and parasympathetic nerve system and as noradrenaline or adrenaline in sympathetic nerve endings. A fuller description of the evidence will be given later for the case of the nerve-muscle junction.

Many other types of synapse have been studied in the central nervous systems of vertebrates and invertebrates (Eccles, 1957, 1964; Furshpan and Potter, 1959; Tauc, 1958; Tauc and Gerschenfeld, 1962) and in smooth muscle (Burnstock and Holman, 1961, 1962), where chemical transmission has been inferred from good, though indirect, evidence, derived mainly from an analysis of the electrical and pharmacological responses of the effector cells. In many of these cases, the identity of the presumed transmitter substance remains unknown, but in some instances it has been possible to show that the electric changes produced by excitatory or inhibitory nerve impulses can be closely imitated by application of minute quantities of specific drugs to the synaptic region of the effector cell. In this way, it has been shown that it is probable that acetylcholine acts as an excitatory transmitter at certain central synapses in vertebrates (Eccles, Fatt, and Koketsu, 1954) and in molluscs (Tauc and Gerschenfeld, 1961; Kerkut and Thomas, 1961) and that the same substance acts as an inhibitory transmitter at other points in the molluscan nervous system (Tauc and Gerschenfeld, 1962). There is also a strong suggestion that γ-aminobutyric acid (see Table 4) may be an inhibitory transmitter to crustacean muscle and that glutamic, or a related amino acid, may possibly be an excitatory transmitting agent at some neuronal, and at crustacean nerve-muscle, junctions (see Kravitz, Kuffler, and Potter, 1963; Takeuchi and Takeuchi, 1964).

8

the transmission of impulses from nerve to muscle

the role of acetylcholine

The neuromuscular junction has been studied in great detail, and much information has been obtained from it which will be helpful in understanding the process of chemical transmission at neuronal synapses generally. Its function is to transfer impulses from the relatively very small motor nerve endings to the large muscle fiber and to cause it to contract. At most of the myoneural junctions in vertebrate muscle, each nerve impulse is followed by a similar impulse in the muscle fibers, which rapidly propagates in both directions toward the tendons, ensuring a sufficiently synchronous activation of the contractile proteins from end to end along the fiber. Thus the vertebrate myoneural junction serves a much simpler purpose than the central synapses of neurons or the peripheral excitatory and inhibitory nerve-muscle contacts of crustacea, where integration of converging signals takes place and where the effect of a single nerve impulse is generally well below the threshold of excitation of the effector cell. To put it somewhat crudely, the vertebrate nerve-muscle junction serves the purpose of a simple relay. One could think of it also as an "impedance matching" device—a kind of pulse transformer whose output provides sufficient electric current to "drive" the low-impedance muscle membrane beyond threshold.

It has already been pointed out that, on structural grounds alone, it is most unlikely that an effective electric cable connection could exist between nerve and muscle. In frog skeletal muscle, the medullated nerve fiber gives off an end bush of terminal nonmyelinated branches of about 1.5-μ diameter that run in shallow grooves of the muscle fiber surface for distances of about 100 μ. All along this terminal course, the nerve establishes synaptic contact with the muscle fiber. In the electron microscope one observes the normal clusters of 500-Å vesicles at numerous places inside the nerve endings (Fig. 27). Presynaptic and postsynaptic membranes are sep-

figure 27

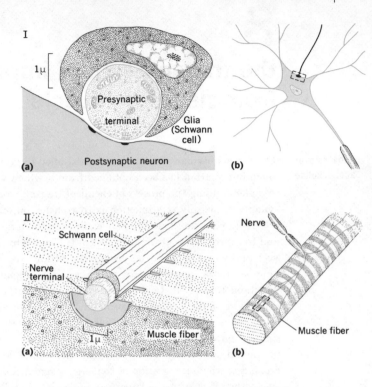

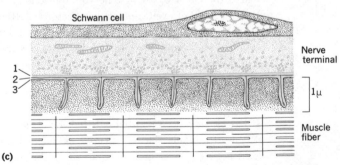

**Diagrams of synaptic structure. Micron scales are only approximate.
I. Neuronal synapse.** (*a*) **Presynaptic: afferent terminal.** (*b*) **A synapse in
relation to other parts of nerve cell. II. Neuromuscular junction of frog.**
(*a*) **One portion of the junction.** (*b*) **General position of endings of motor
axon on muscle fiber, showing portion** (*a*) **as a small rectangle.** (*c*) **Sche-
matic drawing from electron micrographs of a longitudinal section through
the muscle fiber. 1: terminal axon membrane. 2: "basement membrane"
partitioning the gap between nerve and muscle fiber. 3: folded postsynaptic membrane of muscle fiber.**

arated by an extracellular gap containing a basement membrane. The muscle surface is thrown into a regular array of folds which run at right angles to the terminal nerve branch.

Let us consider what the chances are of electric transmission taking place across a typical myoneural junction in one of the largest frog muscle fibers (150-μ diameter). To a brief current pulse, like that produced by a nerve spike, the muscle fiber presents a load (input impedance) of less than 50,000 ohms. To excite the fiber, its resting membrane potential must be lowered from 90 to about 50 mv, which requires a current pulse slightly less than 10^{-6} amp. (It will be seen later that the effect of chemical transmission is to produce a current of about 2 to 3 $\times$ 10^{-6} amp at many end plates, which gives the process an adequate safety factor.)

How much current can the nerve endings supply electrically? Let us take the total length l of the synaptic nerve branches at one end plate as being approximately 1 mm and the "synaptic surface" (which faces the muscle fiber) as $\pi \rho l \approx 2.3 \times 10^{-5}$ cm^2. If the nerve membrane produces an outward pulse whose current density is of the order of 1 ma/cm^2 (the usual value for nonmyelinated nerve and for muscle), this gives a total current of 2.3 $\times$ 10^{-8} amp. Now, even if the whole of this current were to enter the muscle fiber in the synaptic region (i.e., assuming protoplasmic continuity between nerve and muscle) and so were capable of depolarizing the fiber membrane, it could produce a potential change of only 1 to 2 mv. The electrical situation is, however, much worse because of the presence of an extracellular gap of >500 Å and of the post-synaptic membrane impedance (Figs. 26 and 27). If the resistivity of the gap is of the order of 100 ohm-cm, the potential change produced in the gap would amount to only 40 μv. The current entering the muscle fiber would then be reduced to the order of 10^{-11} amp, which would alter its membrane potential by the negligible amount of <1 μv.

In spite of all quantitative uncertainties attached to this argument, it is clear that the structural discontinuity at this synapse renders the possibility of any electric cable transfer extremely unlikely; even if there were protoplasmic continuity, the impedances of nerve terminals and muscle fiber are so badly "mismatched" that one could hardly conceive of a system less suitably designed for electric transmission of signals!

There have been several attempts to test this point experimentally. If a subthreshold current is applied to the nerve near its junction, it produces no detectable local potential change in the muscle fiber (Kuffler, 1949; see also p. 139). When a nerve impulse is set up, it travels down to the ends of the nonmyelinated terminals and starts up an impulse in the muscle fiber. If one places a microelectrode carefully against a point of synaptic contact between nerve and muscle, one records two separate electrical changes (Fig. 28): first, a current pulse generated by the impulse as it arrives in the axon terminal, and then, some 0.5 to 0.8 msec later, another current pulse which arises in the postsynaptic membrane (Katz and Miledi, 1965a and 1965b). The two events are not only separated in time, but the postsynaptic change can be selectively abolished by certain drugs like curare and by lowering the calcium or raising the magnesium concentration. The delay at the myoneural contact points is a consistent and very significant finding; it is a clear indication of an electric discontinuity at the synapse. Evidently, the cable process comes to a halt at the presynaptic terminal, and some other, nonelectrical, process intervenes between the arrival of the nerve impulse and the initiation of an electric signal in the muscle fiber.

The chemical nature of this intermediate process was revealed by the work of Sir Henry Dale and his collaborators (Dale, Feldberg, and Vogt, 1936; Brown, Dale, and Feldberg, 1936), who showed that acetylcholine is released by stimulation of the motor nerve and that this substance has a very potent stimulating action on skeletal muscle. To establish the role of acetylcholine as a chemical transmitter, it has to be shown (1) that its release is from a *presynaptic* site, (2) that its action is at a *postsynaptic* site, and (3) that the amount released by the nerve is sufficient to initiate a muscle impulse.

presynaptic release of acetylcholine

Motor nerve fibers and their endings are known to contain acetylcholine and the enzymic apparatus (choline acetyltransferase) needed to synthesize this substance. The tissue also contains a powerful enzyme which hydrolyzes acetylcholine. This cholinesterase is highly concentrated at the neuromuscular junction, especially on its postsynaptic surface, where its presence can be readily demonstrated by histochemical methods (Koelle and Friedenwald, 1949; Couteaux, 1955). One effect of this hydrolytic

figure 28

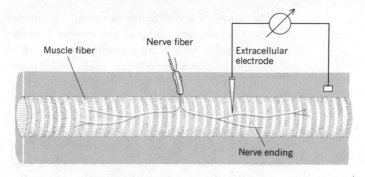

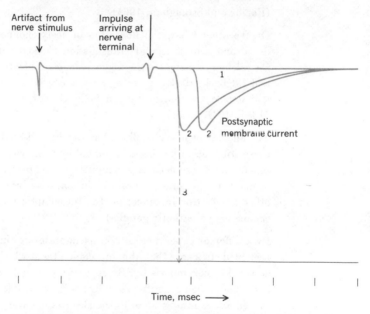

Time, msec ⟶

Focal surface recording from a neuromuscular junction. Under conditions of low calcium and raised magnesium concentrations, the postsynaptic deflection varies between failures (1), and quantal responses (2). Normally, a much larger deflection (3) leads to a muscle spike.

enzyme is that it becomes difficult to demonstrate the release of acetylcholine into the circulating or perfusion fluid because the substance is destroyed before it can reach the collecting vessels. For this reason, an esterase inhibitor (eserine) was used by Dale, Feldberg, and Vogt in their classical perfusion experiments. With this precaution, acetylcholine was detected in the perfusion fluid whenever the nerve was stimulated.

The release of acetylcholine is caused by impulses in the motor axons and not by activity of the muscle. This has been shown in several ways. If one stimulates chronically denervated muscle, no acetylcholine appears (Dale et al., 1936). If one stimulates the motor nerve in the presence of curare, which prevents activation of the muscle fibers, nerve impulses still reach the axon terminals (Katz and Miledi, 1965a) and release the usual amount of acetylcholine (Dale et al., 1936; Emmelin and MacIntosh, 1956; Krnjević and Mitchell, 1961). Even when the muscle fibers have been cut away on either side of the end-plate regions, acetylcholine is still released, provided that the impulses reach the nerve endings (Randić and Straughan, 1964).

On the other hand, the liberation of acetylcholine is greatly reduced and neuromuscular transmission blocked when one lowers the calcium or increases the magnesium concentration (del Castillo and Engbaek, 1954), in spite of the fact that the nerve impulses still invade the motor terminals in the usual way (Katz and Miledi, 1964, 1965c).

The amount of acetylcholine that can be collected during motor nerve stimulation has been estimated by Krnjević and Mitchell to be a few million molecules per impulse per end plate. Similar experiments, with the same general conclusion, have been carried out on other tissues (for instance, on the presynaptic release of acetylcholine in sympathetic ganglia).

By a different experimental approach, an interesting attempt has been made to locate the submicroscopic sites at which acetylcholine is stored in nervous tissue. By separating tissue fractions of brain in the high-speed centrifuge and by assaying them for acetylcholine as well as examining them in the electron microscope, the highest concentration of acetylcholine was found in a fraction containing large numbers of isolated nerve terminals. More recently, this fraction has been analyzed further, and both Whittaker (1964) and de Robertis (1964) have reported that the acetylcholine is stored in the vesicular components of the presynaptic endings.

All this evidence leads to the conclusion that acetylcholine is synthesized and stored in motor nerve terminals, from which it is released by the nerve impulse, and that the subsequent events in the muscle do not add anything significant to this process of release. Calcium ions are needed for this mechanism, whereas curare produces its blocking effect at a later stage of the transmission process, presumably on the postsynaptic side.

postsynaptic action of acetylcholine

One can imitate the action of a nerve impulse in several respects by using a micropipette of the kind described on p. 31, filling it with a fairly strong solution of acetylcholine, and applying the substance ionophoretically to the postsynaptic region of the neuromuscular junction. Very small amounts of acetylcholine are sufficient to depolarize the muscle fiber and to set up impulses, provided that the micropipette is applied to the synaptic region of the fiber surface. Estimates made by several authors (Nastuk, 1953; del Castillo and Katz, 1955a) indicate that 10^{-16} to 10^{-15} mole are enough to excite a muscle fiber in this way. In the normal muscle fiber, only the end-plate region is very sensitive to acetylcholine; as one moves the pipette only a fraction of a millimeter away, much larger amounts are needed to produce a detectable effect and most of the fiber surface seems to be quite insensitive to this kind of chemical stimulus. As will be described later on, this state of locally restricted sensitivity to acetylcholine can be changed experimentally; for example, when the nerve has been cut and allowed to degenerate or after an operative injury to the muscle fibers, the chemical sensitivity spreads along the fiber surface (Thesleff, 1960; Miledi, 1962). During chronic denervation of mammalian muscle, the whole of the fiber may become highly "acetylcholine sensitive." For the moment, the main point of interest is that the excitatory action of acetylcholine occurs in the presence as well as in the absence of the presynaptic axons; the nerve is certainly not required for this effect.

The sensitivity of the muscle to acetylcholine can be greatly reduced by a number of substances, among which curare is the most famous (see Table 4, p. 108). It appears that the curare alkaloids (and many other quaternary ammonium compounds) compete chemically with acetylcholine for its attachment to a reactive membrane molecule (which in the absence of sufficient chemical information is generally classified as a receptor molecule). The process is probably analogous to the competitive inhibition of enzymes, acetylcholine being the normal substrate and curare the competitive inhibitor. If one examines their antagonistic relations quantitatively, they can be fitted reasonably well by the Michaelis-Menten kinetic equations (Jenkinson, 1960). It is important that the neuromuscular blockage produced by curare can be largely or entirely accounted for by its postsynaptic effect, i.e., its interference with the action of acetylcholine. This is consistent with the conclusions reached in the previous section, namely, that curare does not, or does not greatly, affect the presynaptic release of acetylcholine and that its principal site of action must be postsynaptic.

The effectiveness of acetylcholine on the synaptic region of the muscle fiber can be enhanced by a variety of cholinesterase inhibitors. For instance, if one uses a "twin" micropipette, with acetylcholine in one side and a quickly acting cholinesterase inhibitor, tensilon, in the other, a given small dose of acetylcholine produces a much greater and more prolonged depolarization of the muscle fiber if it is "protected" against enzymic hydrolysis by a dose of tensilon from the other pipette. This *potentiation* (i.e., enhancement) of the ACh action is a highly specific effect; it is not observed if, instead of acetylcholine, one uses a stable cholinester like carbachol or decamethonium. These substances also depolarize the end-plate surface, but they are not attacked by the local tissue esterase, and therefore their effect is not potentiated by the esterase inhibitor.

Because of their highly specific potentiating action, it becomes a crucial matter to examine the effect of cholinesterase inhibitors on nerve-muscle transmission. This was done by Brown, Dale, and Feldberg (1936), who showed that the response of a mammalian muscle to a single nerve stimulus becomes larger and longer when eserine is used to inhibit the esterase. The action potential of the muscle becomes repetitive, and the contraction is changed from a "twitch" to a brief "tetanus." However, the interpretation of this finding turned out to be more complicated than it appeared originally. Masland and Wigton (1940) and Feng and Li (1941) showed that in the mammalian nerve-muscle preparation, the effects of eserine and other anticholinesterases are not confined to the muscle fiber and repetitive excitation occurs also in the terminal nerve branches. Thus, the eserine response in the cat presents us with a rather confusing situation, in which both presynaptic and postsynaptic structures are involved, and it becomes quite difficult to ascertain the sites of primary and secondary drug action.

No such difficulty is encountered in the experiments on frog muscle (Feng and Li, 1941; 1951); the principal effect of anticholinesterases, if given in moderate doses, is simply to increase and prolong the postsynaptic depolarization, whether this is produced by a nerve impulse or by applied acetylcholine. No backfiring of motor nerve impulses occurs, but the lengthening of the end-plate potential (e.p.p.), i.e., the postsynaptic potential change, is very striking (Fatt and Katz, 1951).

This is the "pharmacological picture" of the myoneural junction in bare outline. The main features are consistent with the view that acetylcholine acts as transmitter from nerve to muscle. If one examines the drug actions in greater detail, one finds various side effects; for instance, one finds that curare or acetylcholine or eserine in high concentration have also some action on nerve endings and muscle fibers and that a large dose of curare has a slight inhibitory effect on cholinesterase, whereas a large dose of eserine blocks acetylcholine receptors. None of the drugs is "absolutely" specific, but specificity is manifested by the relative concentrations with which the effects are obtained. In this connection, it is not surprising that a substance that competes with acetylcholine for its attachment to an enzyme can, in higher concentration, also compete with it for the attachment to a receptor molecule.

is enough acetylcholine released to stimulate the muscle fiber? This question could not be answered by a simple experiment of the kind Otto Loewi performed on the frog's heart. The reason for this is plain: release and action of acetylcholine in skeletal muscle are highly localized processes and are restricted to a minute fraction of the volume of the perfused tissue. A very small quantity is highly effective immediately after its release so long as it remains concentrated in the small space between nerve and muscle membranes. Diffusion carries it into the external fluid, where it becomes diluted to a very low and relatively ineffectual level, which can be assayed only on a more sensitive preparation (p. 107).

The next best experiment is to compare the estimate of the amount of acetylcholine released by one impulse at one end plate with the amount required for stimulation of a muscle fiber by microapplication to a single end plate. This is, of course, not a fair comparison, for there are bound to be losses when one attempts to collect the acetylcholine by perfusion; and, what is more serious, no method of artificial application has yet been devised that is as efficient as the normal process of release from the nerve endings. A micropipette can be brought close to the most sensitive region of the end plate, but not as close as the presynaptic membrane of the nerve terminal. Furthermore, the release of acetylcholine by the nerve impulse occurs at discrete sites distributed all over the synaptic contact area (p. 131), but the quantity ejected from a fine micropipette tends to flood and saturate the small portion of the end plate that happens to be in closest proximity to the tip of the pipette. The amounts of acetylcholine recovered in perfusion experiments are approximately 5×10^6 molecules per impulse per end plate, whereas the quantities needed to excite a muscle fiber are of the order of 10^7 to 5×10^8 molecules. All one can say is that the difference between these values is not unreasonable; indeed, it is surprisingly small considering the divergent experimental circumstances.

Schematically, neuromuscular transmission involves the following steps:

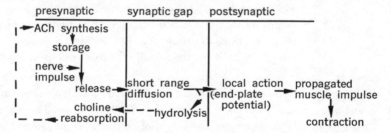

The presence of a special enzyme system in the nerve endings concerned with the acetylation of choline has already been mentioned. It appears that for continuous replenishment of choline, nerve terminals depend largely upon a process that enables them to absorb choline from the extracellular space. This is indicated by the work of Birks and MacIntosh (1957, 1961) on sympathetic ganglia whose acetylcholine content soon becomes exhausted in the course of repetitive stimulation unless they are continuously supplied with choline in the perfusion fluid. A group of substances known as the *hemicholiniums* interferes with the uptake of choline by the nerve ending and so leads to progressive exhaustion of the intracellular acetylcholine store and rapid failure of transmission.

It has been suggested that rapid absorption of choline is brought about by a specific transport mechanism built into the presynaptic membrane and that the postsynaptic hydrolysis of acetylcholine has two important functions—not only does it terminate the local action of the transmitter, but it also provides free choline which can be reabsorbed and resynthesized by the presynaptic terminal.

Of the several stages of transmission indicated schematically above, two have been studied in detail and have yielded quantitative information of general interest. They are (1) the presynaptic mechanism (neurosecretion) by which a nerve impulse enables a specific chemical agent to be released from the cell, and (2) the postsynaptic mechanism by which this substance alters the membrane properties so as to depolarize the fiber sufficiently for a propagated impulse to arise. The latter is a problem which one meets at all chemically operating synapses, and, even more generally, at all those receptor structures (e.g., chemical sense organs) at which a specific substance gives rise to electric membrane changes leading to impulses.

the postsynaptic process: the nature of the end-plate potential

Skeletal muscle fibers are electrically excitable in the same way that nerve fibers are. If one depolarizes the membrane beyond threshold, an impulse is initiated that propagates along the whole fiber in the manner described in Chap. 5. The initial depolarization can be produced artificially (for instance, by passing a sufficient current from an intracellular microelectrode outward through the muscle membrane). This is called *direct* electric stimulation of the muscle, and is in contrast with the normal process of *indirect* activation through the motor nerve. Now, it has been explained (p. 113) that the nerve impulse arriving at the terminals has not enough "power" to depolarize the muscle fiber directly by its action current, and to overcome this impasse, a chemical "mediator," acetylcholine, is secreted from the terminals. After being transferred across the synaptic cleft (by diffusion or possibly a more specific transport mechanism), this substance produces the required local depolarization of the muscle fiber.

Evidence for this view has been obtained by recording the postsynaptic potential changes at the myoneural junction and by comparing the local effect of a nerve impulse with that of locally applied acetylcholine. On arrival of a nerve impulse (frog muscle, 18°C), no electrical change is seen in the muscle fiber for about 0.7 msec, at which time a localized depolarization, the e.p.p., develops rapidly and within 0.5 msec reaches the threshold of excitation (Fig. 29). At this instant, a new action potential arises

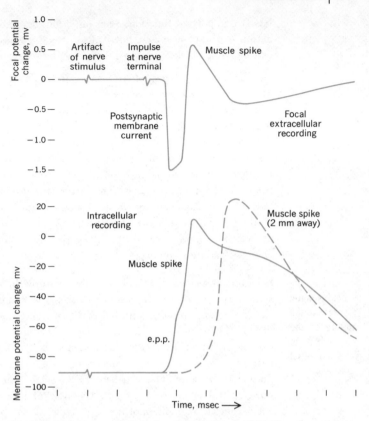

The initiation of a muscle impulse at the myoneural junction. Lower traces show membrane potential change at end plate (solid line) and 2 mm away (broken line). Upper trace (note different voltage scale) indicates approximate time course of focal surface potential changes (see Fatt and Katz, 1951; Katz and Miledi, 1965a).

and travels at constant speed away from the junction. If one gives a small dose of curare, the nerve impulse still reaches the myoneural junction as before, but the subsequent e.p.p. is reduced in size. With a sufficient dose, it fails to reach the excitation threshold and consequently no action potential is elicited in the muscle fiber. If one goes on increasing the amount of curare, the size of the e.p.p. is further diminished until eventually it becomes undetectable. It has already been pointed out that a blocking dose of curare does not affect, or if so only to a minor extent, the release of acetylcholine by the nerve impulse (Dale et al., 1936); but if one applies acetylcholine to the end plate and measures the resulting local depolarization, this is found to be greatly diminished by curare—diminished to nearly the same extent as the e.p.p. (del Castillo and Katz, 1957; Goldsmith, 1963).

Further support has come from experiments with anticholinesterases. Potent inhibitors like prostigmine, eserine, tensilon, etc., cause large increases in amplitude and duration of the e.p.p. as well as of the artificial "acetylcholine potentials" (del Castillo and Katz, 1957; Katz and Thesleff, 1957; Goldsmith, 1963), and there is good quantitative correspondence between the two effects. In view of the chemical specificity of the enzyme and of the low concentrations of inhibitors needed in these experiments, this is strong evidence.

Finally, there are several agents which interfere with the terminal *release* of acetylcholine but which have little immediate influence on the sensitivity of the postsynaptic membrane and do not prevent the invasion of the axon terminal by the nerve impulse. To these agents belong botulinum toxin (Brooks, 1956) and certain changes in the ionic environment (a lowering of calcium and an increasing of magnesium). Under these conditions, the e.p.p. is greatly reduced or abolished, whereas an acetylcholine potential (artificially produced by local application of ACh) shows little or no alteration. The reduction of the e.p.p. at each junction in solutions of low calcium or high magnesium content occurs in an interesting stepwise, or "quantal," fashion, which has revealed an unexpected new feature of the release mechanism (see below).

In view of all these findings, it seems quite safe to conclude that the e.p.p. is produced through a specific action of acetylcholine. The same experiments tell us that this substance is not involved in the subsequent electric events, namely, the initiation and propagation of the muscle spike. To check this point, one keeps the microelectrode in the muscle fiber at the end-plate region and applies alternate stimuli to the nerve and to the muscle fiber directly. Curare or anticholinesterases in moderate doses, which profoundly change the electric response to nerve impulses, have no effect on the size and rate of rise of the muscle spike produced by a directly applied current and do not alter the threshold level or the direct subthreshold potentials produced by an applied current pulse.

time course of transmitter action

Having satisfied ourselves that the primary potential change that a nerve impulse sets up in a muscle fiber is due to the action of acetylcholine, the question arises of what physicochemical process underlies this effect.

In curarized muscle, the e.p.p. has a simple wave form: it rises in about 1 msec and lasts about 20 msec. It spreads along a few millimeters of the fiber surface, and, like any subthreshold potential change, becomes distorted and attenuated by the leaky cable properties of the muscle fiber. The time course and spatial spread of the e.p.p. have been analyzed, and it has been shown that after the first few milliseconds the potential change represents a passive decline governed simply by the cable constants of the muscle fiber and by the rate at which electric charge is distributed along and dissipated across the fiber surface (Eccles, Katz, and Kuffler, 1941; Kuffler, 1942; Katz, 1948; Fatt and Katz, 1951; Takeuchi and Takeuchi, 1959; Falk and Fatt, 1964).

The initial active phase, during which the transmitter reacts with the postsynaptic membrane and causes it to become depolarized, lasts about 5 msec, most of the activity being confined to the first 2 to 3 msec. These figures apply to normal and curarized muscle; after treatment with an anticholinesterase, the active period lasts much longer, and the transmitter causes the local depolarization to be maintained for as long as 100 msec. Under these conditions, the amount of acetylcholine released by the impulse (which is about 10^{-17} mole) causes an electric charge of approximately 10^{-7} coul to flow across the postsynaptic membrane (a total flux of at least 10^{-12} moles of univalent ions).

How is this very large amplification of local current (and of ionic flux) brought about? To put the answer in simple terms, acetylcholine reacts with receptor molecules in the postsynaptic membrane and alters the properties of the membrane so that it becomes highly permeable to small cations (for example, Na^+, K^+, Ca^{++}, NH_4^+, and a number of quaternary ammonium R_4N^+ ions). The effect is accompanied by a lowering of the membrane resistance and a flow of ionic current through the "activated" surface area. The intensity of the effect increases with the local concentration of acetylcholine and of the available receptor molecules. It is therefore greatest when a given quantity of acetylcholine is applied to the receptors at very close range, when local enzymic hydrolysis has been prevented, and, of course, when there is no competitive agent like curare blocking the access of acetylcholine to the receptors.

The depolarization (e.g., in the form of the e.p.p.) that acetylcholine normally produces is caused by an inward flow of sodium ions, but the permeability to potassium is increased at the same time, and the resulting efflux of potassium prevents the e.p.p. from moving beyond the zero-potential level. In fact, the e.p.p. (and the underlying ion current) reverse sign when the membrane potential of the muscle fiber is displaced beyond 10 to 20 mv, negative inside. In practice, this can be done most simply by performing a "collision" experiment in which a muscle spike, set up by direct stimulation, serves to displace the membrane potential from −90 to +35 mv. In addition, an impulse is set up in the nerve and made to arrive at the end plate and liberate acetylcholine at selected moments during the passage of the directly excited action potential (del Castillo and Katz, 1954). In this way, the null point of the e.p.p. was found to be at −10 to −20 mv. Below that level (i.e , nearer the resting potential), acetylcholine causes net current to flow *inward* through the membrane and therefore to depolarize the fiber; above that level, the net current flows *outward* and the potential change is in the reverse direction from the normal e.p.p. These conclusions have been confirmed in several other experiments (for instance, experiments that displaced the membrane potential with steady current and applied acetylcholine artificially (Axelsson and Thesleff, 1959) and experiments using a voltage-clamp method (p. 81) to determine the net ionic current flow directly (Takeuchi and Takeuchi, 1960).

The reversal point for the end-plate current (about −15 mv) differs very significantly from the "sodium equilibrium" potential E_{Na} (approximately +50 mv). To interpret this finding, the electrical membrane model of Fig. 16 is helpful. The null point of the e.p.p. does not correspond to the equilibrium potential of any single one of the three principal ionic channels, but it could be explained if several channels, for example, Na *and* K, or Na, K, and Cl, are opened up simultaneously by the transmitter action. This problem was studied carefully by Dr. and Mrs. Takeuchi (1960) in experiments in which they changed the three ion concentrations in the medium separately and determined the effect on the position of the null point. The conclusion was that the transmitter, acetylcholine, raises the permeability to Na and K ions simultaneously and to about the same extent, whereas it produces little or no change in the chloride permeability of the end plate.

Another important finding was that the ionic permeability or conductance change produced by the transmitter is independent of the membrane potential of the muscle fiber (Fatt and Katz, 1951; Takeuchi and Takeuchi, 1960). In other words, a given quantity of acetylcholine produces a local current flow whose intensity is directly proportional to $(E - 15)$ mv, where E is the p.d. (potential difference) across the membrane, outside minus inside. This again distinguishes the process underlying chemical transmitter action from that of electric excitation in which the ionic permeability change is critically dependent on the level of the membrane potential (and so can become regenerative).

The electrical effect of acetylcholine on the motor end plate has been likened to a "shunt" or "short-circuit" placed across the membrane. This is a fairly apt description because normally the transmitter drives the membrane potential toward a depolarized low value which corresponds roughly to the diffusion potential one might obtain if the membrane had suffered a localized "breakdown." Actually, we now know that the rise of ion permeability of the active end-plate surface is not entirely indiscriminate, but it is almost nonselective between small cations. It could be pictured as a formation of leaky ionic channels whose "protein lining" retains fixed negative charges and so rejects the passage of anions.

In frog muscle, the release of the transmitter certainly produces a powerful short-circuiting effect. It quickly depolarizes the muscle membrane beyond the threshold of excitation, and during the ensuing spike, it even opposes the reversal of the membrane potential. Electric recordings from the active end-plate region show a complicated sequence of potential changes (Fig. 29). They are the resultant of two interacting processes: (1) the transmitter action (simultaneous rise of Na and K conductances), which tends to displace the membrane potential toward -15 mv and to hold it there for 1 to 2 msec and (2) the action potential (sequential rise of Na conductance, then of K conductance), which tends to rise quickly toward $+50$ mv and then to return to the resting level.

The two events occur in adjacent parts of the same cell membrane and produce a composite effect which can be analyzed and separated into its components by the previously mentioned "collision experiments." The membrane resistance has also been measured during these changes. It was found that the transmitter produces a very large increment of the membrane conductance that is separate from, and in *addition* to, that occurring during a directly evoked spike. The electrical effect of the transmitter is indeed equivalent to that of a transient membrane "puncture" opening up a pathway of 2 to 3×10^{-5}/ohm conductance (Fatt and Katz, 1951; del Castillo and Katz, 1954c).

9

quantal nature of chemical transmission

spontaneous
release of
acetylcholine;
a quantal
process of
neurosecretion

One of the conclusions drawn from the preceding chapter is that the synaptic region of the muscle fiber membrane is an extremely sensitive "detector" for small quantities of acetylcholine. Its specialized properties can be revealed by the microelectrode recording technique even without using any form of stimulation at all. In 1950, Fatt and Katz observed that in isolated, "resting," muscle the junctional region is the site of spontaneous discharges of minute e.p.p.'s that are about 0.5 mv in amplitude and occur at random moments at an average frequency of about one per sec.

Individual discharges originate at sharply localized focal points scattered along the synaptic axon terminals. The electrical changes are equivalent to a momentary local increase of membrane conductance of approximately 10^{-7}/ohm and an associated inward pulse of ionic current of about 10^{-8} amp (del Castillo and Katz, 1956b; Takeuchi and Takeuchi, 1960b). The amplitude of the resulting potential change varies with the size of the muscle fiber. The smaller the fiber, the higher its input impedance and, therefore, the larger the depolarization produced by a given pulse of current (Katz and Thesleff, 1957a).

Except for their spontaneous random occurrence and their small size, the discharges are indistinguishable from the e.p.p.'s produced by nerve impulses; for example, curare suppresses them and cholinesterase inhibitors enhance their amplitude and duration with the same doses and to approximately the same extent. They are called *miniature* end-plate potentials (Fatt and Katz, 1952), and there is very little doubt that they arise from localized impacts of small quantities of acetylcholine upon the postsynaptic membrane. The phenomenon has been observed at all kinds of vertebrate myoneural junctions, and similar spontaneous potentials have also been found to occur at neuronal synapses in the central nervous system where the chemical transmitters have not yet been identified (Katz and Miledi, 1963). Normally, the miniature e.p.p.'s are all well below the "firing level" of the muscle fiber and so remain localized and produce no contraction. But when their amplitude has been enhanced by cholinesterase inhibitors, they occasionally rise in some fibers above the excitation threshold and then lead to visible spontaneous twitching.

Although all these effects are recorded postsynaptically in the muscle fiber, it is clear that the muscle end plate merely serves as a sensitive detector for a process of acetylcholine secretion which originates in the motor nerve endings. The evidence for this comes from several findings. First, the spontaneous local activity disappears some days after the motor nerve has been cut—at the same time that the nerve endings disintegrate.* Second, botulinum toxin, which irreversibly prevents the release of acetylcholine from the nerve endings, also abolishes the miniature e.p.p.'s (Brooks, 1956; Thesleff, 1960). Finally, the frequency of the discharges is controlled directly by the membrane potential of the nerve terminals but not by the potential of the muscle fiber (del Castillo and Katz, 1954).

To summarize, there is very strong evidence that the motor nerve terminals are, even "at rest," in a state of intermittent "secretory activity" and that they liberate small quantities of acetylcholine at random intervals at an average rate of about one per sec. A nerve impulse causes this activity to become enormously intensified for a very brief moment so that a few hundred of these unitary events become synchronized within less than one millisecond.†

---

* In the frog, this period is followed later by a resumption of spontaneous discharges at very low rate. This is associated with, and possibly caused by, local proliferation of terminal Schwann cells which establish "synaptic contacts" with the muscle fiber (Birks, Katz, and Miledi, 1960; Miledi and Slater, 1963).

† The membrane conductance change associated with each of these events is restricted to a very small area (a few square microns; see Katz and Miledi, 1965a). It follows that the affected area of the postsynaptic membrane must undergo a very intense change of ionic permeability. If 10 μ^2 are uniformly affected, then—for a value of $\Delta g = 10^{-7}$/ohm (del Castillo and Katz, 1956; Takeuchi and Takeuchi, 1960b)—the membrane resistance R_m of the affected area would be as low as 1 ohm-cm². The area may be even smaller, and the effect more intense. [The theoretical limit is set by the convergence resistance presented by a small "hole" in the membrane ($R_m = 0$). With a surrounding medium of specific resistance 100 ohm-cm, a hole of 0.1-μ size would present a resistance of approximately 10^7 ohms.]

There has naturally been a good deal of speculation concerning the possible *function* of the spontaneous microsecretion of transmitter from the nerve endings. It has been suggested, for instance, that the mysterious "trophic" influence by which the motor nerve cell regulates the excitability and the metabolism of its subordinate muscle fibers is mediated by the continued secretion of acetylcholine even in the absence of nerve impulses. But the evidence is not altogether in favor of this idea (Miledi, 1963). All one can really say at present is that some of the transmitter substance that is continuously being built up and accumulated in the nerve terminals "spills over" into the synaptic interspace and in doing so produces small but detectable postsynaptic potential changes.

The question arose of whether the spontaneous discharges are due to acetylcholine leakage by diffusion, one molecule at a time, from the nerve endings. This was quickly ruled out when the effects of locally applied acetylcholine were tested. A small dose of acetylcholine, whether it is applied to the end plate by ionophoresis or applied diffusely in the muscle bath, causes a local depolarization whose size is continuously graded according to the dose and whose time course varies with the distance and speed of application. The potentials evoked by one or a few molecules of acetylcholine are evidently far below the resolving power of the recording method, and one must conclude that discrete potential changes like the miniature e.p.p.'s, with their regular size and time course, can only arise from a synchronous action of a packet of acetylcholine containing a large number (perhaps thousands) of molecules at a time. Moreover, the packet must be highly concentrated and delivered at a very short distance from the receptors, for the time course of the reaction (i.e., of the current pulse) that it produces is very brief and not compatible with a diffusion path of more than about a micron.

We are dealing here not with a "molecular overspill," but with a quantal spontaneous release, in which concentrated multimolecular packets of acetylcholine are secreted at random moments, in all-or-none fashion, from discrete points of the terminal axon membrane. These are all-or-none events at the subcellular level; they are quite different from the action potential, which is a quantal response involving one cell at a time.

It was thought that small regions of the terminal nerve branches might "fire" spontaneously—perhaps triggered into electric activity by random fluctuations in their membrane potential—without necessarily causing an impulse to propagate into the larger branches of the axon (Fatt and Katz, 1950). However, this was difficult to reconcile with the observation that spontaneous miniature e.p.p.'s that arise at adjacent spots of a single axon terminal (say 10 to 15 μ apart) are not synchronized, as they would be if they were caused by a local action potential, but are quite independent of one another (Katz and Miledi, 1965a). In any case, this explanation was ruled out when it was found that the spontaneous end-plate activity persists even when nerves and muscles have been depolarized in a potassium-rich solution and deprived of external sodium so that all electric excitability was eliminated (del Castillo and Katz, 1955b).

Another proposition was that the quantal release might be due to the activation of a specific molecule, acting as a kind of "acetylcholine gate" in the presynaptic membrane, which opens for a moment and allows a certain amount of acetylcholine to escape. This has not been ruled out, but there are arguments which make this idea appear weak. According to this explanation, the *size* of the acetylcholine quantum is governed by the duration of a process in the axon membrane, namely, the interval during which the gate is open or during which an "acetylcholine carrier molecule" is in an activated state. Now, the experiments of del Castillo and Katz (1954a), Boyd and Martin (1956), Martin (1955), Liley (1956), and Katz and Miledi (1965b and 1965c) have shown clearly that the size of the acetylcholine packet is not altered by the membrane change associated with the nerve impulse. What *is* altered is the frequency, or probability of occurrence, of the quantal event (this goes up by a factor of several hundred thousand). Similarly, depolarization of the nerve terminals, produced by applied current, increases the frequency but does not alter the amplitude of the miniature e.p.p.'s. Thus, the acetylcholine quantum remains constant in spite of widely varying conditions of the cell membrane from which it is released. This made the hypothesis of a controlling membrane "gate" or "carrier system" unattractive and suggested that one had better look for a cell component other than the surface membrane when trying to find a structural counterpart of the miniature e.p.p.

At this stage the characteristic presynaptic "vesicles" were revealed by the electron microscope, and the suggestion naturally arose that they could be the subcellular particles in which the transmitter is stored and from which it is released in a quantal all-or-none fashion. It seemed conceivable that critical collisions between vesicle and axon surface could cause their membranes to "break" and so cause the vesicular contents to be discharged into the synaptic gap.

The rate of such reaction would depend on two factors: (1) the collision frequency and (2) the number of reactive molecules in the vesicular and axon membranes. The enormous rise in secretion rate during the impulse could be explained if the number of reactive sites of the axon membrane increases tenfold for a 15-mv depolarization (Liley, 1956b).

the quantal composition of the end-plate potential

The present picture depends to a large extent upon one basic finding, namely, that the spontaneous miniature e.p.p. and the underlying membrane conductance change is the basic unit of transmitter action and that the large e.p.p. that results from a nerve impulse is made up of an integral multiple of such unit components.

Convincing evidence was obtained when it became clear that the number of such components contributing to the response at a single myoneural junction can be varied by altering the external magnesium and calcium concentrations. Calcium is an essential "cofactor"; without it, a depolarization of the nerve endings fails to increase the rate of acetylcholine secretion. Magnesium competes with calcium and acts as an inhibitor of this process.

If one lowers the normal calcium concentration and adds magnesium to the muscle bath, the amount of acetylcholine delivered by an impulse can be reduced to a very low level, and under these experimental conditions, the statistical composition of the end-plate response becomes immediately apparent. The e.p.p. is reduced *in steps*, which correspond to the dropping out of individual miniature units. When the responding units are small in number, e.p.p.'s evoked by successive impulses show a marked random fluctuation in amplitude with occasional total failures of response.

A statistical analysis of such responses was carried out by several groups of investigators, and it was found that the distribution of amplitudes is fitted accurately by a *Poisson series*, whose "unit class" is identical with the spontaneously occurring miniature potentials.

Let us illustrate this by an example (Boyd and Martin, 1956). Recordings were made from a single end plate—first, of a series of 78 spontaneous miniature e.p.p.'s and then of 198 responses to single nerve impulses repeated at intervals of several seconds. The amplitudes of all potentials were measured and are represented in the histograms of Fig. 30. The mean size of the spontaneous potentials is 0.4 mv, with a standard deviation of ±0.086 mv. The amplitudes of individual responses fluctuated to a much greater extent. There were 18 complete failures, and the rest ranged from 0.3 to 3.0 mv in size. Their distribution shows a number of peaks clearly defined at 0.4, 0.8, and 1.2 mv. The mean size of all responses (including the 18 failures) was 0.933 mv, that is, 2.33 times the mean spontaneous potential.

These are the "raw" data. In applying Poisson's law, we are testing the validity of the following assumptions: (1) that each response is made up of an integral number (0,1,2,3,4, etc.) of units whose mean size and variance are identical with the mean size and variance of the spontaneous potentials, and (2) that each "unit response" (i.e., the release of any one packet) is an event of very low statistical probability p, where $p \ll 1$. In other words, each time a nerve impulse arrives at the terminals, it causes the release of a few acetylcholine packets out of a very large available population; the chance of any one unit being released remains small at all times and is not contingent upon the release of any other member of the population.

If these assumptions are correct, Poisson's theorem should apply. This theorem tells us how many of our 198 impulses are likely to release one, two, three, or more packets of acetylcholine and how many are likely to release nothing at all. Poisson's law tells us, in fact, that if the *mean* number of packets liberated by an impulse is m, then the chance p of observing any particular number x (0,1,2,3, etc.) is

$$p_x = \frac{m^x}{x!} e^{-m}$$

For a sufficiently large number of observations N (which in our case is 198), the value Np_x should come close to the actually observed number of responses which contain x quanta and which are consequently made up of a summation of x miniature e.p.p.'s.*

Thus if we know the mean number m of quantal components released by an impulse, we can calculate the number of responses containing $0,1,2,3, \ldots x$ quantal components. Now, using assumption (1), we express the mean value m in our series of 198 responses by

9† $$m = \frac{\text{mean amplitude of response}}{\text{mean amplitude of spontaneous e.p.p.'s}} = \frac{0.933 \text{ mv}}{0.4 \text{ mv}} = 2.33$$

The Poisson theorem then predicts that our responses should be distributed as follows:

$n_0 = 198e^{-m} = 19;$ observed   18

$n_1 = mn_0 \quad = 44$ $(44)^a$

$n_2 = \dfrac{m}{2} n_1 \quad = 52$ (55)

$n_3 = \dfrac{m}{3} n_2 \quad = 40$ (36)

$n_4 = \dfrac{m}{4} n_3 \quad = 24$ (25)

$n_5 = \dfrac{m}{5} n_4 \quad = 11$ (12)

$n_6 = \dfrac{m}{6} n_5 \quad = 5$ (5)

$n_7 = \dfrac{m}{7} n_6 \quad = 2$ (2)

$n_8 = \dfrac{m}{8} n_7 \quad = 1$ (1)

$n_9 = \dfrac{m}{9} n_8 \quad = 0$ (0)

[a] The figures in parentheses are subject to small errors; they were obtained by dividing the histogram of Fig. 30 into successive groups centered around amplitudes of multiples of 0.4 mv.

---

* There appear two different kinds of "numbers" in this form of analysis which must not be confused: (1) the number x of quanta released by an impulse and (2) the number n_x of impulses releasing x quanta.

† This simple equation can only be used provided that m is small and the response does not exceed a few millivolts in size. For larger responses, a correction must be applied because, unlike quantal conductance changes, miniature potentials do not add linearly beyond a limited range. To allow for this effect, the right-hand side of Eq. (9) has to be multiplied by the factor $1/(1 - v/75)$, where v is the mean amplitude of the response in mv (see Martin, 1955).

The number of failures (n_0) provides a simple and direct test of the theory. All one has to do is count numbers of successes and failures to respond, and determine the *mean* amplitudes of evoked and spontaneous potentials (a safe and accurate procedure when dealing with a large series of observations). This gives us two independent means of determining m: from Poisson's law we get

10 $$e^{-m} = \frac{n_0}{N} = \frac{\text{no. of failures}}{\text{no. of impulses}}$$

If we combine this with equation (9), we obtain

11 $$\frac{\text{Mean size of response}}{\text{Mean size of spontaneous e.p.p.'s}} = \ln \frac{\text{no. of impulses}}{\text{no. of failures}}$$

In the present example, from Eq. (9) $m = 0.933 \text{ mv}/0.4 \text{ mv} = 2.33$, whereas from Eq. (10), $m = \ln 198/18 = 2.4$

Equation (11) has been tested over a wide range by several investigators with frog and mammalian nerve-muscle preparations and in all cases excellent agreement was found (del Castillo and Katz, 1954a; Boyd and Martin, 1956; Liley, 1956).

The Poisson formula can also be applied to the complete amplitude histogram of Fig. 30. This is a little more complicated because the size of the miniature "unit potential" itself varies somewhat and the larger the number x of such unit components adding up to an evoked potential, the greater must be the statistical variation of the observed amplitudes. However, to translate the Poisson numbers (that is, $n_1, n_2, n_3 \ldots n_x$) into an amplitude histogram is not at all difficult; one simply has to follow a clear-cut statistical prescription, which is illustrated in Fig. 31. We construct a separate histogram for each Poisson class (of quantum number x) and then add them together. The separate histograms are defined by three parameters. The total number to be distributed is n_x, the mean amplitude is vx, where v is equal to the mean amplitude of spontaneous potentials, and the variance is $\sigma^2 x$, where σ is the standard deviation of the miniature e.p.p. (assuming a normal size distribution).

Figures 30 and 31 are examples of the result and the analysis of an experiment by Boyd and Martin (1956). The procedure has been described here in detail because the result of this statistical analysis

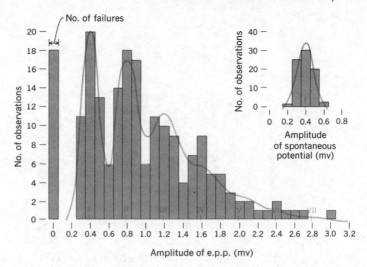

Histograms of e.p.p. and spontaneous potential amplitudes (inset), from a mammalian end plate. Peaks of e.p.p. amplitude distribution occur at 1, 2, 3, and 4 times the mean amplitude of the spontaneous miniature potentials. A Gaussian curve has been fitted to the latter and used to calculate the theoretical distribution of e.p.p. amplitudes. Arrows indicate expected number of failures (zero amplitude). (From Boyd and Martin, 1956.)

enables one to state with complete confidence (1) that the miniature e.p.p. represents the unit of subcellular action at the nerve-muscle synapse and (2) that the quantum of ACh release remains unchanged whether it occurs spontaneously during periods of undisturbed rest of the motor axon or at the peak of activity of the axon membrane when the impulse arrives at the motor nerve endings.

the release of acetylcholine— an electrically controlled form of neurosecretion

The terminal effect of a nerve impulse is to produce a large increase in the rate of a secretory process that goes on spontaneously all the time and reveals itself by the appearance of postsynaptic potential changes. The miniature e.p.p.'s can be used as a sensitive indicator of the rate at which secretion of acetylcholine packets proceeds, and a study of the factors which control the frequency of the miniature e.p.p.'s is likely to throw light on the mechanism of this process.

One of the significant findings was that depolarizing the nerve endings by applied current or by raising the potassium concentration produces a graded increase of the discharge rate (del Castillo

figure 31

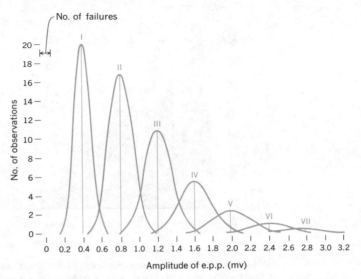

Method of obtaining the continuous curve in Fig. 30. A Poisson distribution was calculated for a mean value m (mean amplitude of e.p.p. responses)/(mean amplitude of spontaneous potentials). The calculated numbers of each Poisson class have been distributed along Gaussian curves corresponding to multiples of the spontaneous potentials (see Fig. 30). Algebraic summation of ordinates gives the continuous curve of Fig. 30. (From Boyd and Martin, 1956.)

and Katz, 1954b; Katz, 1958, 1962). The effect has been followed quantitatively by Liley (1956b), who concluded that the frequency of the miniature e.p.p.'s rises exponentially by a factor of 10 for a depolarization of 15 mv. Liley pointed out that the production of the normal e.p.p., that is, the release of a few hundred quantal units within a fraction of a msec, would be explained if the exponential relationship holds throughout the rise and fall of the terminal axon spike and if the release follows the presynaptic potential change without time lag.

Calcium and magnesium alter the exponential constant. Calcium increases, and magnesium reduces, the effect of a given depolarization (see del Castillo and Katz, 1954), which explains their influence on ACh release by nerve impulses. Liley's hypothesis has many attractive features, but it rests on a rather long extrapolation from findings which cover only a relatively small range of potential changes. It is certain that depolarization is a controlling factor in the process of ACh release, but the quantities and time relations involved require further study.*

These experiments yielded an important by-product. By passing electric current through the terminal portion of the nerve, one can depolarize the endings sufficiently to raise the output of acetylcholine and the frequency of the miniature e.p.p.'s one hundred times or more (which, according to Liley's assay, requires a depolarization of over 30 mv). Yet not a trace of the presynaptic steady potential change is transmitted to the muscle fiber; all that one records are the miniature e.p.p.'s whose frequency goes up during the current flow. Observations of this kind show very clearly the special properties of the neuromuscular junction, where cable transmission has been totally replaced by quantal secretion of a chemical transmitter. Its rate of release is electrically controlled in the nerve ending, and it then depolarizes the postsynaptic membrane by specific chemical action.

cumulative effects of repetitive nerve impulses

We have so far confined the discussion to the elementary processes associated with the arrival and transmission of a single motor nerve impulse. It is one of the distinguishing features of a synapse that, unlike the relative constancy of the axon impulse, its "power of transmission" is subject to very large variations, many of which are caused by slowly subsiding aftereffects from previous impulses. For instance, in a curarized frog muscle one often observes that the e.p.p.'s evoked by repetitive nerve impulses at first grow in amplitude (the second e.p.p. of a series may be nearly twice as large as the first), reach a maximum after 6 to 10 volleys, and then progressively decline in size. The initial growth of individual e.p.p.'s (Fig. 32) is called "facilitation," whereas the progressive decline goes under various names like "neuromuscular depression" or "Wedenski inhibition." Another well-known phenomenon is the so-called "postactivity potentiation," which is a long-lasting increase of transmitting power of single impulses observed *after* a period of intense nerve activity. These are important modifications of the synaptic process, and can cause the size of the e.p.p. to vary over a more than tenfold range. A statistical analysis of the

---

* The recent work of Katz and Miledi (1965*b*) has shown that there is, in fact, a measurable time lag between the arrival of the action potential and the transmitter release.

figure 32

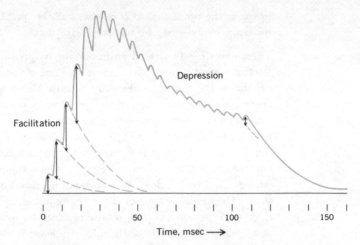

Progressive changes of postsynaptic potentials (for example, e.p.p.'s) during repetitive impulse bombardment, illustrating "facilitation" followed by "depression."

kind described on p. 134 has shown that the site of action is presynaptic and that the changes in the size of the e.p.p. are due to a larger or smaller *number* of acetylcholine quanta being released without change in the unit size. It is possible that relatively small alterations in the amplitude of the nerve spike or local changes in the ionized calcium concentration could produce large alterations in the amount of transmitter released.

Del Castillo and Katz (1956*a*), in reviewing the situation, pointed out that all the experimental changes in ACh output which had been produced so far were modifications in the number, not in the size, of the quantal packets. They suggested, however, that it might be possible to reduce the quantum *size* by interfering with the intracellular mechanism of ACh synthesis.

It has been proposed that ACh may be synthesized within the nerve endings by particle *A* (microsomes) while it is accumulated and stored in particle *B* (perhaps vesicles), from which it is released in an all-or-none fashion. Suppose a "vesicle" accumulates ACh from a low level in the cytoplasmic environment to a much higher concentration ready for release. This would be a very effective mechanism for releasing a large amount from a focal point of the terminal axon membrane. The vesicular concentration of ACh would, however, depend on the level in the surroundings (just as the K concentration of a muscle fiber depends on that of the external medium). Suppose the process of intravesicular accumulation works at a speed and efficacy comparable to that of potassium accumulation by a muscle cell; then, if it takes a muscle fiber of 100 μ some hours to equilibrate, a 500-Å vesicle would require only a few seconds. On this basis, one might expect the size of the ACh quanta and miniature e.p.p.'s to depend on continuous intracellular synthesis and to fall as the existing intracellular store becomes depleted. There are a number of agents (glucose deprivation, blockage of choline uptake by hemicholinium, compound HC3) that are said to interfere with ACh synthesis in vivo. These agents were tested on the frog and mammalian neuromuscular junction by several investigators (Martin and Orkand, 1961; Thies and Brooks, 1961), but until quite recently, the results were negative, i.e., they failed to show any reduction in quantum size. A positive finding has been reported by Elmqvist, Quastel, and Thesleff (1963). Using small doses of HC3, they found that the miniature e.p.p. gradually diminished in amplitude during prolonged nerve stimulation, whereas the statistical composition of the e.p.p. (the number of contributing units) remained unchanged.

10
transmission of signals across neuronal synapses

The vertebrate nerve-muscle junction has provided a good deal of information that will help in guiding us through the far more complex behavior of synapses in the central nervous system. Most of our knowledge of central synapses comes from the study of mammalian motoneurons in the spinal cord of the cat (Eccles, 1957, 1961, 1964). It is very probable that many of the synaptic connections of these motor nerve cells operate by a chemical transmitter mechanism. It is certain that some of the postsynaptic potential changes arise from alterations in ionic permeabilities and have a characteristic reversal point (null point) similar to that of the e.p.p. Furthermore, there is evidence for a "quantal release" of excitatory and inhibitory transmitters that produces spontaneous and evoked potentials similar to miniature e.p.p.'s (Katz and Miledi, 1963). This behavior strongly suggests chemical transmitter action, but until the substances have been identified, the point cannot be regarded as finally established.

The main functional difference between the nerve-muscle junction and most neuronal junctions in the central nervous system is that the former operates as a simple relay by which an impulse is transmitted without fail and with minimum delay from a single nerve cell to a large number of muscle fibers, whereas neuronal synapses are used, in general, to transcribe impulses that arrive in the presynaptic terminals into graded subthreshold potential changes of the next neuronal membrane. This difference is of a *quantitative* kind. It could be explained by the fact that the size of the synaptic contact area between two individual neurons is, in general, much smaller than the motor end plate. The membrane of a central neurone is the principal site where "integration" takes place of messages converging onto it from many other nerve cells, some producing excitatory, others inhibitory, effects. In the present chapter we will discuss the mechanisms by which the integration of converging input signals is brought about.

Let us recall some simple "general principles." First, excitatory and inhibitory nerve impulses are all alike; their antagonistic effects depend solely upon the special properties of their synaptic connections. Secondly, all processes of integration within the post-synaptic cell must be confined to a *subthreshold* range of variations of the membrane potential. The neuronal membrane can "handle" any number of local potential changes, and add or subtract them, so long as the resulting sum total does not exceed the threshold level. When this is reached, an impulse is triggered which propagates along the axon and momentarily cancels any other incoming messages. Thus, reception and integration of signals is a local, graded process by which the membrane potential of a nerve cell is moved, or is prevented from moving, toward the firing level. Unlike the impulse, which is an all-or-none signal designed to propagate with ample safety margin and great stability of amplitude, neuronal integration operates at the subthreshold levels of the membrane potential.

There is evidence (Eccles, 1957; Eyzaguirre and Kuffler, 1955; Grundfest, 1957; Furshpan and Furukawa, 1962) that in many nerve cells the points of signal reception are spatially separated from that of impulse initiation, the latter being at the axon origin and the former being located on the cell body and dendrites. Moreover, dendrites and cell body appear to be regions of relatively low electric excitability. Their threshold is high, and this provides the cell membrane with a relatively wide range of operating levels for local subliminal changes.

the crustacean nerve-muscle junction The vertebrate nerve-muscle junction provides us with insight into a chemical transmission process similar to those operating very probably at many central synapses, but it lacks the special organization of the central neuron, with its multiple, converging and antagonistic, input signals. An interesting model, which fits much more closely, is found in the neuromuscular system of crustacea (Wiersma, 1941). Here, individual muscle fibers are innervated by multiple excitatory and inhibitory axons whose endings converge on to many regions of the muscle membrane. The force and speed of the muscular contraction are the final resultant of these converging, and antagonistic, nerve signals, just as the impulse discharge of a motor axon is the final outcome of multiple synaptic influences impinging on its central cell body.

The study of the crustacean nerve-muscle system, with its peripheral integrative mechanisms, has contributed a great deal to our understanding of central synaptic processes (Wiersma, 1941; Fatt and Katz, 1953; Dudel and Kuffler, 1961a to 1961c) and, because of its simple synaptic organization, will serve as a useful introduction to the problems of central nervous activity. Some crustacean muscles, e.g., the opener muscle of the crayfish claw, present a particularly simple type of "dual innervation," all the fibers being supplied by branches of two antagonistic axons, one of which evokes contraction and one of which prevents contraction. Most *vertebrate* fibers are innervated in a single microscopic region, the motor end plate, which is situated in the middle; a new impulse is set up at this point, which then propagates in both directions toward the tendinous ends of the muscle and secondarily excites the contractile apparatus in the interior of each fiber (see Chap. 11). *Crustacean* muscle fibers, however, do not depend on a self-propagating impulse mechanism. Many of them are not capable of producing full-sized all-or-none action potentials of the kind occurring in axons or vertebrate muscle. In this respect (in the inability to produce propagating all-or-none spikes of ample safety margin), crustacean muscle fibers have a poorly developed electrical excitability (see above, p. 95). They depend instead on a distributed supply of nerve endings scattered all along the fiber surface, which produce a simultaneous electrical change that acts as a graded local stimulus to the contractile apparatus. This distributed innervation enables the muscle to dispense with a propagating mechanism of its own; the nerve impulse reaches the whole of the fiber surface at practically the same time and can, therefore, evoke a synchronous and effective development of muscular tension. Moreover, because of the absence of an all-or-none response, the contraction of each fiber is subject to gradation by the summating effects of successive nerve impulses, which reinforce one another, and by the antagonistic interaction of the two axons. Thus, a crustacean muscle fiber possesses to a considerable extent the integrative capacity that characterizes a central neuron (which the skeletal muscle fibers of vertebrates do not have).

We are not concerned, at this stage, with the chain of events by which the depolarization of the surface membrane leads to contraction in the interior of a muscle fiber. This will be considered in a later chapter (p. 163). The relevant questions at the moment are how excitatory and inhibitory nerve fibers exert their opposite effects on the postsynaptic membrane and what kind of interaction takes place between them.

When the *excitatory* axon to a crustacean muscle is stimulated, one finds that a single nerve impulse produces only a very small depolarization in the muscle fiber, and perhaps no visible contraction at all. The potential change resembles the e.p.p. seen in deeply curarized vertebrate muscles, with the difference that it is not localized in one region but occurs from end to end along the muscle fiber. During repetitive stimulation, say with a battery of 20 nerve impulses at a rate of 50/sec, the successive potential changes rapidly increase in amplitude (facilitation, see page 139) and build up to a large depolarization of the muscle membrane. This is accompanied by a gradual rise of tension. The rate at which these distributed "e.p.p.'s" are built up is governed by the frequency of the incoming nerve impulses and, in turn, regulates the speed and force of the ensuing contraction.

If one stimulates the *inhibitory* axon, the effect is quite different: the contraction suddenly stops; the muscle relaxes as though excitatory nerve impulses had been switched off, although in fact both axons are being stimulated simultaneously and continue to discharge their impulses.

"Inhibition" is one of the most striking synaptic events whose mechanism has mystified physiologists for generations, but has been greatly clarified by recent studies, especially those of Eccles and his collaborators (Coombs, Eccles, and Fatt, 1955; Eccles, 1957, 1961a, 1964). It is known that there are at least two different microscopic sites on which the inhibitory action is exerted, one in the presynaptic terminals of the excitor axon and the other at the postsynaptic membrane of the effector cell, and that the inhibitory nerve impulse can interfere with several discrete links of the excitatory chain (Eccles, 1961a; Frank and Fuortes, 1957; Frank, 1959). In these respects, the properties of the crustacean nerve-muscle contacts closely resemble those of central synaptic connections (Kuffler, 1960; Dudel and Kuffler, 1961c).

postsynaptic effects

When a transmitter substance like acetylcholine is released from a nerve terminal and reacts locally with the postsynaptic cell, it produces an increase of ionic conductance, or permeability. This statement is true in a very general way; it applies not only to the vertebrate nerve-muscle junction at which ACh acts as excitatory transmitter but also to the pacemaker region of the heart, where ACh released by vagal nerve impulses produces *inhibition* of the heart. It applies also to many central synapses where acetylcholine and other, unidentified transmitter substances are released and produce excitatory or inhibitory effects (see Tauc, 1958; Tauc and Gerschenfeld, 1962; Kerkut and Thomas, 1964). At the crustacean nerve-muscle junctions the excitatory transmitter substance is unknown, but there are good indications that the inhibitory substance is γ-aminobutyric acid (Kravitz et al., 1963). It is present in relatively high concentrations inside the inhibitory (but not in the excitatory) nerve fiber, and—if artificially applied—produces all the known inhibitory effects.

The essential difference between an excitatory (E) and inhibitory (I) action on the postsynaptic membrane can be stated in very simple terms: the E effect causes a depolarization; the membrane potential is driven to, or beyond, the threshold level at which action potentials (and/or contractions) arise. The I effect causes the membrane potential to be stabilized at (or to move toward) a *subthreshold* level at which no active response (spike or contraction) can arise. Both effects are produced by an increase of ionic permeability; the difference lies in the particular "ionic gates" that are being operated by the excitatory and inhibitory transmitter action.

To appreciate this point, we consult once more the three-channel circuit diagram previously shown in Fig. 16. Suppose an active response occurs when the membrane p.d. is reduced to -50 mv from its resting level of -70 mv. This can be achieved by a chemically induced increase of ionic permeability, but *only* if the Na channel is included. Without this, and without the resultant inward current of Na ions, it would not be possible to obtain the rapid membrane depolarization needed for the excitatory response. If a transmitter agent caused an opening of only K or Cl channels, this would tend to stabilize the membrane potential at or near the resting level, and so lead to inhibition.* The effect would be rather

---

* Inhibition is often accompanied by a moderate "hyperpolarization," i.e., an increase of the membrane p.d. beyond the initial level. This is a consequence of the fact that normally the membrane is not wholly impermeable to Na ions, so that a selective opening of the K channel leads to hyperpolarization by moving the membrane potential closer to E_K.

similar to that occurring during the refractory period of the squid axon, after an impulse has been discharged (see p. 86), when—to put it rather crudely—the Na gates are firmly shut and the K gates kept wide open.

The scheme of Fig. 16 has been used to illustrate, in a general way, how opposite effects may be produced by similar conductance changes operating on different ionic channels. It should be noted, however, that there are many cases (including the excitatory junctions of crustacean muscle) in which the specific channels have yet to be identified. It is possible that other ions, not represented in Fig. 16 (for example, Ca or Mg) may make an important contribution to synaptic current flow in some situations.

Much evidence has accumulated to confirm the view of a *common ionic mechanism* underlying synaptic excitation and inhibition. The final effects are of opposite sign in the two cases and the membrane potential may be displaced in opposite directions, but this results simply from a selection of different ionic channels, whose conductances are being raised by the transmitter action. In the heart, ACh produces hyperpolarization and inhibits the rhythmic beat because it raises the K permeability alone (or at least predominantly), driving the membrane toward −80 mv; at the motor end plate, ACh causes depolarization and gives rise to a muscle impulse because both K *and* Na permeabilities are simultaneously increased, driving the membrane toward −15 mv. Similar conductance changes probably underlie the effects that excitatory nerve impulses produce in the crustacean muscle fiber and in the spinal motoneuron, whereas the antagonistic, inhibitory effects in these cells are due to a selective, or predominant, increase of the chloride permeability (Coombs et al., 1955; Boistel and Fatt, 1958).

facilitation

One of the characteristic properties of crustacean nerve-muscle systems (and of many central nervous connections) is that the efficacy of excitatory impulses increases greatly with repetition. This process is known as *facilitation*, and it is due to a combination of two factors. First, there is the summation of successive potential changes in the postsynaptic membrane, each impulse producing a subthreshold depolarization that adds to the remainder of the preceding potential changes. A more important factor, however, is that the amount of transmitter released by each impulse increases during a repetitive series. The phenomenon observed in *normal* crustacean muscle is very similar to that obtained in a vertebrate muscle that has been exposed to a high magnesium and low calcium concentration. Furthermore, Dudel and Kuffler (1961*b*) have shown that the same quantal release mechanism is involved. They discovered spontaneous "junction potentials" in crayfish muscle (see also Dudel and Orkand, 1960), analogous to the miniature e.p.p.'s, and they found, through the statistical analysis described on p. 134, that the evoked response is made up of integral multiples of such unit potentials and that their numbers are statistically predictable by Poisson's law. During a train of nerve impulses, the *number* of units contributing to individual responses increases progressively, indicating that the nerve impulse becomes more and more effective in releasing quanta of transmitter substance.

presynaptic inhibition

In the course of their investigation, Dudel and Kuffler (1961*c*) made the unexpected discovery that an *inhibitory* nerve impulse, quite apart from directly influencing the ionic permeability of the crustacean muscle membrane (p. 147), was able to interfere with the release of the excitatory transmitter by its antagonistic axon. This process has become known as "presynaptic inhibition," which implies that there is some kind of interaction going on between inhibitory and excitatory nerve endings that is probably dependent upon the presence of a special synaptic connection between them.

The experimental finding was that the number of unit potentials (excitatory) produced in the muscle fiber was greatly reduced when an impulse in the inhibitory axon preceded the excitatory nerve impulse by a few milliseconds. It is possible that inhibitory axons send out terminal branches to contact the excitatory nerve branches, as well as the muscle fiber directly, and that the same transmitter, possibly γ-aminobutyric acid, is released at both kinds of contact. If it selectively increased Cl permeability at both sites of action, not only would it tend to stabilize the membrane potential of the muscle fiber and counteract any depolarizing influence, but by a similar action it would tend to reduce the amplitude of the nerve spike in the excitatory endings and so reduce the efficacy of the terminal release (see p. 138; see also Dudel, 1962; Liley, 1956*b*).

The importance of these findings is that they brought to light an unexpected mechanism of synaptic interaction, which now appears to be of very widespread occurrence in the central nervous system (Eccles, 1961a). One may suspect that presynaptic interactions of different signs exist (facilitation, or "reduction of inhibition," as well as inhibition itself), and that they might be important not only for short-term signaling but in establishing long-term "conditioning" of nervous pathways (cf. p. 157).

Let us sum up our present knowledge of the crustacean neuromuscular synapses. Excitatory nerve impulses lead to a quantal release of a transmitter substance that raises the ionic permeability (probably to sodium and other cations) and depolarizes the muscle membrane, causing contraction. Above a certain level, the depolarization may become regenerative and cause a more intense and faster contraction. However, the muscle fibers do not in general give all-or-none spikes or require a propagating impulse mechanism, as they are innervated "all over."

Crustacean muscle fibers have, in addition, an inhibitory nerve supply. Inhibitory impulses release a transmitter substance (possibly γ-aminobutyrate) that has two discrete effects. (1) It acts on the muscle fiber directly, raising its chloride permeability and stabilizing or repolarizing the membrane potential. (2) It acts on the terminal (or preterminal) excitatory nerve branches so as to reduce the amplitude of the impulse and, indirectly, the liberation of the transmitter (Dudel and Kuffler, 1961c; Dudel, 1962).

Both inhibitory mechanisms cause the effect of excitatory nerve impulses to be greatly diminished and so interfere with the activation of the contractile mechanism.*

central neurons Our knowledge of the basic mechanisms at the synapses of central neurons has been greatly advanced since the advent of the intracellular recording technique; it is largely derived from studies on mammalian spinal motoneurons (Eccles, 1957, 1964; Fatt, 1957; Frank and Fuortes, 1957).

---

* There remains the possibility of a third site of inhibitory action, namely, on the chain of events by which depolarization causes contraction. There are some indications that such an additional action may occur (Hoyle and Wiersma, 1958), and the present summary statement may well be incomplete.

The elementary processes at these synapses are not very different from those already discussed, but their organization and spatial distribution over the surface of the effector neuron and its dendritic branches are far more complex and add another degree of freedom to the integrating capacity of the nerve cell.

It is now widely accepted that the site of origin of the efferent impulse is near the point of emergence of the axon from the cell body (the so-called axon hillock, or the "initial segment" of the nerve fiber). This appears to be brought about by a large gradient of electric excitability within the neuronal membrane; the threshold is lowest at the point of axon origin, is considerably higher in the cell body and large dendrites, and increases to the point of inexcitability in the more remote branches of the dendritic system. The latter conclusion is based on postulates and plausible predictions rather than direct evidence. Indeed, without invoking special local membrane properties, it is difficult to see what useful contribution the fine terminal dendrites can make to the integrative function of the neuron.

Terminal dendrites may be as much as 1 mm away from the soma and axon hillock. The diameter of the distal branches is of the order of one or a few microns—over 10 times less than the size of the cell body. There is evidence that the synaptic action on central neurons occurs in the "quantal" fashion and that the effects of spontaneous transmitter release may depolarize the cell body as much as 1 to 2 mv (Katz and Miledi, 1963; cf. Kuno, 1964). The local depolarization, produced by spontaneous release at a terminal dendritic synapse, is likely to be very much larger because the voltage change is inversely related to the cell size and increases with the "input impedance" of the cable structure (Katz and Thesleff, 1957a; p. 99). The cell body presents an input impedance of only a few megohms; the tip of a fine dendritic branch, as much as 100 megohms. The terminal dendrites are therefore likely to be subjected to large spontaneous potential changes and would tend to discharge impulses and impair the stability and integrative function of the whole neuron, unless their excitation threshold were very high.

On the other hand, if they are to act merely as passive leaky cables, with a specific membrane resistance of a few thousand ohm-cm^2 (as found in the cell body), a synaptic potential change originating in them would be attenuated so much that no appreciable influence could reach the critical sites near the axon hillock. The situation presents a puzzle that has not yet been properly resolved. It may be that the dendritic membrane resistance, as well as the excitation threshold, increases with distance from the cell body.

A motor nerve cell will fire an impulse (and elicit a twitch in the peripherally connected muscle fibers) when the balance of excitatory and inhibitory impulses arriving in its presynaptic terminals is sufficient to depolarize the axon hillock by 15 to 20 mv. With an electrode implanted in the cell body, one records then a series of inflections (Fig. 33): first, the subthreshold postsynaptic potential and then a sudden stepwise increase of the depolarization due to the initiation of an impulse at the most excitable site—the point of origin of the axon. When this reaches the "soma threshold," a second stepwise increase occurs, which is due to a regenerative spike developing in the membrane of the cell body—close to the site of recording. This is the view reached by Fuortes, Frank, and Becker (1957) and Eccles (1957) on the basis of a careful analysis of the three components and their time relations; it is widely accepted, though alternative interpretations have been advanced (see Fatt, 1957a and 1957b).

The initial depolarization (which is known as the excitatory postsynaptic potential, or e.p.s.p.) has been likened to the e.p.p. in

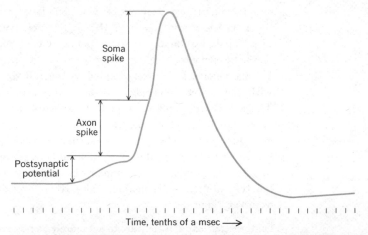

figure 33

The synaptic initiation of a motor nerve impulse due to strong afferent "monosynaptic" excitation. Intracellular recording with a microelectrode in the cell body of the motor neuron.

skeletal muscle. There are a number of analogies, and it is probable that the underlying ionic mechanisms are similar. Thus, the reversal point of the e.p.s.p. (see p. 125) is in the neighborhood of complete depolarization (zero p.d. across the cell membrane), which is not far from the equilibrum level of the e.p.p. It cannot be determined with the same degree of accuracy because the synaptic depolarization originates at many points scattered over the dendrites as well as the cell body, and the electrical method used to displace the membrane potential does not affect all these regions uniformly. In these circumstances, one tends to find a reversal point that is a little too far from the resting potential—farther than the "true" equilibrium level (see Burke and Ginsborg, 1956).

central inhibition
As in the crustacean nerve-muscle system, at least two different kinds of inhibitory action have been found in the synaptic connections of spinal motoneurons.

The initial observations of Eccles and his colleagues (Brock, Coombs, and Eccles, 1952) indicated that synaptic inhibition could be accounted for by a hyperpolarization, i.e., an increase of the membrane potential induced by the action of an inhibitory transmitter substance. This potential change is called the inhibitory postsynaptic potential (or i.p.s.p.). The i.p.s.p. subtracts from any synaptic depolarization and makes it correspondingly more difficult to drive the neuronal membrane potential toward the firing level. It turned out subsequently that the i.p.s.p. has a reversal point which is only 10 mv higher than the resting potential of the motoneuron and which is greatly influenced by the chloride concentration inside the cell. Diffusion of Cl ions from a KCl-filled microelectrode inserted into the neuron is sufficient to cause a reversal of sign of the i.p.s.p. from hyperpolarization to depolarization (Coombs, Eccles, and Fatt, 1955). An extensive study of the effects of various anions has shown that not only Cl but practically all anions below a certain hydrated size influence the amplitude of the i.p.s.p. and can cause it to reverse if they are injected ionophoretically into the interior of the nerve cell. The general conclusion from these experiments is that the inhibitory transmitter "opens the gate" to chloride and other negatively charged ions of the same and smaller size. In this way, the membrane potential tends to be moved toward, and clamped at, the Cl equilibrium potential, which is normally near the resting level or at a slightly more negative level. The more depolarized the membrane, the stronger will be the influx of Cl (tending to restore the potential and move it away from the firing level). The effect is very similar to the direct inhibitory action of nerve impulses on crustacean muscle fibers.

A further analogy to the crustacean nerve-muscle system came to light when it was found that the postsynaptic influence could not account for the whole of the inhibitory effects of afferent nerve impulses on motoneurons (Frank and Fuortes, 1957; Eccles, 1961a). In both systems, a suitably timed inhibitory impulse will greatly reduce the e.p.s.p. (depolarization) evoked by a subsequent excitatory impulse. The effect in the spinal cord is usually much more intense and persistent than would be explicable merely by the postsynaptic change in chloride permeability. Moreover, the reduction is evident even when the membrane p.d. of the effector cell is artificially raised well beyond the chloride equilibrium. Under these conditions, the i.p.s.p. itself becomes a depolarization, and yet the total postsynaptic response is greatly reduced by the inhibitory impulse. This can be explained by a presynaptic interaction similar to that which has been demonstrated for the crustacean system by Dudel and Kuffler (1961c).

E_{Cl} about 5 mV more(-) than R.P.

Eccles has found a very consistent correlation of three phenomena that seem to be invariably associated. When a specific pathway of inhibitory nerve fibers is stimulated, it produces a long-lasting *depolarization* in the *excitatory* nerve endings. This is accompanied by a lowering of the electrical threshold of the terminal part of the excitatory axons and by a striking reduction of the e.p.s.p. that they produce in the effector neuron. The probable explanation for this inhibitory "syndrome" is as follows. The inhibitory nerve endings exert a synaptic influence, not only on the effector cell but also on the presynaptic excitatory terminals. This "presynaptic action" produces an ionic permeability change and partial depolarization, which in turn gives rise to increased local excitability but causes the amplitude of the presynaptic spike to diminish and so reduces the quantal release of excitatory transmitter. There are numerous analogies from other junctions for each individual link in this chain of events; but the detailed mechanism of presynaptic inhibition still remains to be worked out. It will be of particular interest to find the reversal point of the presynaptic depolarization and to learn what kind of ionic permeability change is involved.*

In addition to these two inhibitory processes, whose widespread occurrence has been established by a large body of evidence, other kinds of inhibitory mechanisms have been postulated over the years and one of these, namely, the *direct electrical*, or *ephaptic*, type, has been shown to exist in the special case of the Mauthner cell (Furukawa and Furshpan, 1963; see p. 105). It is quite probable that other varieties and combinations of inhibitory processes will come to light as the detailed exploration of different kinds of nervous synapses proceeds.

It is of interest that a theory of inhibition that was very widely discussed 50 years ago has found little support in modern investigations. This was an attempt to explain central inhibitory processes in terms of a peripheral phenomenon known as *Wedenski inhibition*. This is an intense depression of neuromuscular transmission that develops if impulses are fired into the myoneural junction in too rapid succession. From this analogy, it has been argued that one and the same afferent axon could be used to excite or inhibit an effector neuron, depending simply on the rate at which impulses are discharged in it. It is doubtful whether this kind of process, namely, "depression by excessive use," plays an important role in normal synaptic integration. As an experimental phenomenon, however, it has been of considerable interest to many authors, and, indeed, there is still some discussion concerning the different contributing factors (see Rosenblueth, 1950).

Wedenski inhibition can result from postsynaptic as well as presynaptic failure. Nerve fibers can carry impulses at a rather higher frequency than muscle fibers; the excitability of the axon recovers

---

* It could be an increase of Cl permeability, like that at the postsynaptic inhibitory site, but to explain the depolarization and excitability rise, one would have to assume an unusually low chloride ratio for the excitatory nerve endings. Alternatively, the permeability change might be similar to that underlying the e.p.s.p., but this seems even less probable. In any case, it would seem that this presynaptic effect could very easily lead to the discharge of additional excitatory impulses. (It has, indeed, been suggested that the so-called "dorsal root reflexes" are an example of this kind.) Thus, there remains at present the puzzling phenomenon that a depolarizing action which can bring the excitatory nerve endings close to their unstable firing level appears to be used for the purpose of producing a powerful and stable inhibitory effect.

at a faster rate, or, in other words, the motor nerve has a shorter refractory period than the muscle. If a nerve impulse reaches the end plate while the muscle fiber is still refractory, it will simply produce an e.p.p. locally. This keeps the muscle membrane depolarized during the refractory period, and it further delays the restoration of its normal excitability and ionic permeability (see page 86). The arrival of more nerve impulses in sufficiently rapid succession will maintain the local depolarization and so, instead of eliciting muscle impulses, will perpetuate the state of inexcitability. This is one of the factors that can lead to a Wedenski depression.

Other factors involve the motor nerve and its endings. Krnjević and Miledi (1958) have shown that there are regions of low safety margin at intramuscular points of nerve branching at which blockage of the impulse tends to occur during high-frequency stimulation. Furthermore, during a repetitive impulse bombardment at high frequency, the acetylcholine release mechanism—after an initial period of enhancement (facilitation)—tends to fail progressively, so that after about 10 to 20 impulses not enough transmitter may be released to excite the muscle fiber. Finally, under special conditions (e.g., when anticholinesterases are being used), there is the possibility that so much acetylcholine may accumulate that the end-plate receptors themselves become refractory (or chemically desensitized) and fail to maintain the local depolarization. This last factor has so far been demonstrated convincingly only by prolonged artificial drug application (Thesleff, 1955; Katz and Thesleff, 1957c); whether the localized and brief transmitter release effected by a series of nerve impulses can lead to a sufficient accumulation is still uncertain.

Finally, it is theoretically possible that nerve impulses might produce synaptic inhibition by releasing a substance which competes with the excitatory transmitter. This is a process well-known in enzyme chemistry as *competitive inhibition;* the inhibitor molecule is not destroyed or transformed, but by attaching itself to the receptive group of the enzyme, it competitively displaces the substrate molecule and so blocks the normal enzymic reaction. This kind of mechanism underlies the action of certain blocking drugs. For instance, curarine competes with acetylcholine for its attachment to the end-plate receptors and so abolishes the transmission of the nerve impulse. There is, however, so far no evidence that a similar competitive block is involved in synaptic inhibition. It is conceivable that in specific cases antagonistic axons might converge on to the same microscopic region of an effector cell and interact in this way, but experimentally this occurrence has not been demonstrated.

central facilitation As in the peripheral nerve-muscle system, the efficacy of a nerve impulse in releasing transmitter from the axon terminals can become greatly enhanced as a result of repetitive activity. Such phenomena are grouped under the names of *facilitation* (meaning that each impulse facilitates the transmission of the next one) and *postactivation potentiation* (the potency of impulse transmission being greatly enhanced after a prolonged period of impulse activity). The interesting feature about these processes is that the change is confined usually to the terminals that had been carrying impulses and does not spread to other synapses on the same effector neuron. Thus, if a neuron is supplied by, say, 10 converging excitatory axons, and axon *A* has been subjected to repetitive bombardment, only this axon will show a greater power of transmission during the subsequent period of facilitation; the other synaptic connections will not be affected.

This restrictive factor distinguishes the simple process of facilitation from the much more complex mechanism of *conditioning,* in which the successful association of impulses in *two* converging pathways facilitates the subsequent transmission along one of them alone. We are still quite ignorant of the cellular mechanisms that underlie the long-term changes involved in conditioning and "learning," and, in fact, we are still searching for adequate analytical methods that will allow us to approach this problem. There is a remarkable gulf between our understanding of the brief events in nerve and muscle cells (impulse conduction, synaptic transmission, muscle contraction) and our ignorance of the important long-term changes which occur in nervous pathways, which are the basis of "memory" and underlie the formation of new functional connections.

There are two cellular sites at which long-term synaptic changes are likely to take place. (1) *Postsynaptically*, the sensitivity of the cell membrane to a transmitter substance can vary over a wide range. This has been shown experimentally for skeletal muscle, whose sensitivity to acetylcholine can be greatly increased by denervation or transection (Thesleff, 1960; Miledi, 1960a, 1962, 1963; Katz and Miledi, 1964) and reduced by reinnervation (Miledi, 1960b). Presumably, these changes depend upon chemical alterations of the surface membrane of the cell, and it is very likely that the protein structure of the cell surface is influenced in some way by the other cells with which it makes a synaptic connection. (2) *Presynaptically*, the release of the transmitter by an impulse is equally variable and depends on a whole series of dynamic properties. The rate of synthesis, the distribution and storage of transmitter substances within the terminals, the efficacy of the release mechanism by the terminal membrane—all these are factors which depend on the specific protein metabolism of the cell and factors upon which long-term changes could operate. Various interesting suggestions have been made concerning the physicochemical feedback mechanism by which a series of impulses could influence the protein and nucleic acid metabolism of the cell, but in its present state the field is too obscure to make detailed speculations profitable.

11
initiation of
muscle contraction

In the previous chapters, when the properties of the cell membrane
were discussed, nerve and muscle fibers were treated for practical
purposes as identical, and the experimental evidence obtained
from either of them was presented as almost interchangeable. It
is true that the fast "twitch fibers" of vertebrate skeletal muscle
closely resemble nerve axons (in particular, the nonmyelinated
variety of axons) in their ability to produce action potentials at
any point and to propagate them in either direction from end to
end. In both cases, the surface membrane of the cell possesses a
special mechanism by which it is able to transmit electric signals
rapidly and without fail and in this way cause excitation to spread
very quickly over the whole of the cell. In nerve, this process
serves the obvious purpose of communicating a signal to a remote
point, e.g., at the other end of a long peripheral axon. In muscle,
the action potential, traveling at a speed of a few meters per second, serves to produce sufficiently quick "mobilization" of the
contractile apparatus in the interior of the cell.

To produce effective mechanical force, all parts of the muscle fiber
must develop active tension simultaneously. Suppose a muscle
fiber 5 cm long is innervated at a single end plate in the middle of
its length and produces impulses traveling at a speed of 5 m/sec.
Each impulse initiates a twitch whose tension rises to a peak in,
say, 30 msec and then falls 50% in about the same time. The
excitation delay between the middle of the fiber and its two ends
is only 5 msec, which produces only a slight phase lag in the tension
development and does not seriously reduce the force exerted at the
tendon.

In some long muscle fibers, this phase lag is further diminished by
the provision of two or three discrete end plates spaced at 1- to
2-cm intervals along the fiber. As the impulse in the myelinated
motor nerve travels much faster than the subsequent action poten-

tial in the muscle fiber, the provision of multiple end plates further improves the synchronization of the contraction.

In many invertebrate animals, propagation of an action potential along muscle fibers is dispensed with and a synchronous activation of the whole fiber is brought about by an extreme case of multiple innervation, motor nerve endings being distributed at many points along the muscle fiber. The necessity for such an arrangement seems to have arisen in these animals for an entirely different reason, namely, to obtain fine control and gradation of muscular activity with a minimum number of motor nerve channels. Most arthropod muscles (e.g., the big muscles of the lobster claw) are supplied by very few (some by only one) motor axons, plus an inhibitor axon. (Both are nonmyelinated fibers and are found among the largest peripheral axons, so achieving the necessary speed of conduction; see p. 92.) If each muscle fiber had been supplied with only one or two localized end plates and therefore had to produce its own propagated impulse to spread activity, the whole muscle could give only a triggered all-or-none response to each motor nerve signal. Since the fiber has a distributed innervation all over its surface, however, the need for a triggered muscle impulse does not exist, and this type of impulse has been replaced by a nonpropagated, graded form of electric response similar to the e.p.p. (see p. 146), whose amplitude is controlled by the frequency of successive nerve impulses and by interaction of the motor with the inhibitory nerve fiber.

Many frog muscles contain a proportion of fibers whose electrical and mechanical responses resemble those of crustacean muscle and are quite distinct from the twitch fibers which constitute the major part of skeletal muscles. This is the so-called *tonic*, or *slow fiber*, system which is characterized by a very slow development of tension in response to repeated nerve impulses. The muscle fibers differ in their permeability properties from those in the twitch system; their resting potential is relatively low (60 mv as against 90 mv), and they are unable to produce a regenerative type of action potential. Like crustacean muscle fibers, they receive scattered innervation with junctions distributed along the whole length. The nerve impulses (confined to a special set of small-diameter axons) produce a graded depolarization that is similar in many ways to the e.p.p. (Kuffler and Vaughan Williams, 1953;

Burke and Ginsborg, 1956) and that arises, like the e.p.p., from a release of discrete packets of acetylcholine all along the nerve endings.

In all these muscle fibers, however, a displacement of the resting membrane potential in the direction of depolarization, whether local and graded or propagated and all-or-none, is invariably the stimulus which starts the chain of events leading to the development of tension and to muscle contraction.

The mechanism of contraction itself will not be described here. There have been many striking advances in this field which deserve to be dealt with in a separate book (see Huxley, A. F., 1957, 1964; Huxley, H. E., 1960). After transmission of the nerve impulse, energy is liberated by the muscle fibers in the form of heat and mechanical work, whose quantities and time relations have been measured and analyzed with very great precision by A. V. Hill. Hill (1938, 1956) has shown that the energy released by an impulse is not a preset constant quantity, but varies in a characteristic fashion with the force against which the muscle pulls. It appears that there is an automatic mechanism by which the force, or tension, on the muscle regulates the rate of liberation of its chemical energy. During a prolonged steady contraction, energy release varies linearly with b ($P_0 - P$), where b is a characteristic rate or velocity constant of the muscle, P_0 is the maximum force which the muscle can hold, and P is the actual force against which it shortens.

The active shortening of muscle fibers is brought about by the interaction and movement of two different kinds of protein filaments, described by F. B. Straub and by A. Szent-Györgyi (1947) as actin and myosin. New and fascinating clues to the action of these contractile proteins have been provided by the electron-microscope studies of H. E. Huxley (1957, 1963). Hanson and Huxley (1955, 1957) found that muscle fibers contain two types of protein filaments—thick ones, which consist of myosin, and thin ones, made of actin (Figs. 34 and 35). Each thick filament is made of a stack of long L-shaped myosin molecules (H. E. Huxley, 1963), whose side pieces can interact and form temporary cross-linkages with adjacent actin filaments. The two types of protein form two regular arrays of filaments that overlap and "interdigitate" to a variable extent (Fig. 35); when the muscle is being

(a)

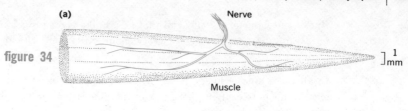

Nerve

figure 34

$]\frac{1}{mm}$

Muscle

(b)

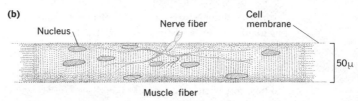

Nucleus

Nerve fiber

Cell membrane

$]50\mu$

Muscle fiber

(c)

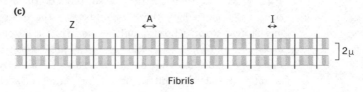

Z   A   I

$]2\mu$

Fibrils

(d)

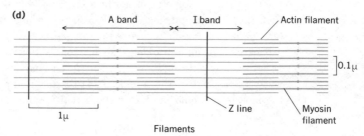

A band   I band   Actin filament

$]0.1\mu$

1μ Z line   Myosin filament

Filaments

(e)

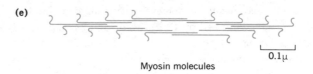

0.1μ

Myosin molecules

Structural organization of vertebrate striated muscle.

stretched, the two arrays tend to be pulled apart like two pieces of a telescope; during shortening of the muscle fiber, the two arrays slide into one another. It appears that, during activity, cross-links between myosin and actin filaments are made and broken many times in rapid succession and that the reactive groups on the protein molecules are arranged spatially in such a way that a directional movement of the two filaments toward one another occurs, which results in rapid shortening of the whole muscle or in the development of active tension.

Our knowledge of the physical chemistry of the contractile process is still in a fragmentary state. It appears that the crucial chemical reaction associated with active shortening is the splitting of ATP by an enzymic branch of the myosin molecule, and that relaxation occurs when this process is reversed by resynthesis of ATP.

The problem that is more closely connected with our present theme is: how is the contractile system excited? What are the intermediate steps by which the action potential, or, more generally, the local depolarization, of the cell membrane stimulates the contractile protein filaments and elicits the release of mechanical energy?

Here again, a number of interesting, though so far scattered, clues have appeared in the recent literature. It is clear that depolariza-

figure 35

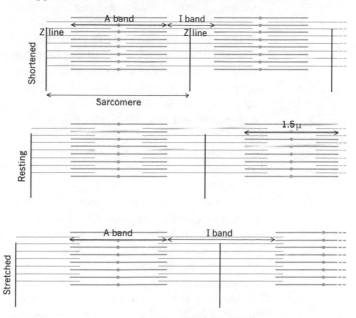

I band: Actin (thin) filaments (about 1μ long) on either side of Z line.

A band: Myosin (thick) filaments (about 1.5μ long) + partially overlapping actin filaments.

Diagram illustrating the "sliding-filament theory" of muscular movement. The structure is characteristic of vertebrate skeletal muscle (see also Fig. 34).

tion of the surface membrane is the usual stimulus for contraction; it is a necessary precursor, but not a sufficient condition. In an ionic environment containing about 2-mM calcium, a muscle fiber starts to develop tension when its membrane is depolarized from, say, 90 to 50 mv, and will develop nearly maximum tension when the membrane potential is reduced to 40 mv (Hodgkin and Horowicz, 1960). If the membrane potential is lowered suddenly and maintained at a low level, e.g., by adding potassium to the muscle bath, the tension develops rapidly to a maximum plateau and then slowly declines. The contractile mechanism adapts or "accommodates" to the persistent electrical change in a way that resembles the "inactivation" of the regenerative excitation process of the surface membrane (p. 85).

In several types of muscle, the presence of calcium was found to be essential for the contractile process. This is particularly clear in frog's heart muscle, in which the contractile effect of a depolarization (e.g., of the action potential) is promptly and reversibly abolished by removing calcium from the bath. Lüttgau and Niedergerke (1958) have shown that the range of membrane potentials in which contraction of the heart can be shifted in either direction by altering the external ion concentration—in particular, that of calcium and sodium. Calcium is an essential "cofactor" in initiating the contraction of the heart; sodium is a "competitive inhibitor" and antagonizes the calcium effect. The higher the Ca/Na ratio, the less depolarization is needed to initiate the contractile response; with a sufficiently high value of Ca/Na, the heart muscle fibers contract even at the normal level of the resting potential.

The precise point of action of calcium is still uncertain. If one homogenizes muscle tissue and subjects it to differential centrifugation, a particulate fraction can be prepared that contains the vesicular fragments of what is known as the *endoplasmic reticulum*. (The latter is an intracellular network of fine tubes that is believed to transmit stimuli from the cell surface to the contractile structures inside.) It is of great interest that calcium is actively accumulated and stored in vitro by these vesicles (Hasselbach and Makinose, 1961; Ebashi and Lipmann, 1962; Weber, Herz and Reiss, 1963).

It is certain that some special mechanism is required to conduct the activating stimulus from the surface membrane to the protein filaments in the center. Diffusion of a chemical agent from the surface to the middle would be too slow, and it is more likely that a special conducting apparatus exists that brings the electrical stimulus provided by the action potential closer to the center. It is possible that the tubes of the reticulum form an electrical extension of the surface membrane and so enable the potential change to travel inward (see Franzini-Armstrong and Porter, 1964). That this may be so is indicated by a recent analysis of the electric capacity of the muscle fiber, which is several times larger than that of nonmyelinated axons of similar size (Falk and Fatt, 1964). It appears that the membrane capacity of muscle is made up of two parallel components. One is about $2~\mu f/cm^2$ and corresponds to the ordinary axon membrane covering the whole fiber; this, however, is paralleled by another capacitative channel of about $5~\mu f$, which contains a small series resistance. The latter value may correspond to the extra capacity provided by the tubular walls of the reticulum, and the resistance possibly arises in the narrow tubular channels and their connections with the external fluid.

The work of A. F. Huxley and R. E. Taylor (1958) has thrown further interesting light on the existence of a special electric path from the surface to the contractile apparatus. They found that if one applies highly localized electric stimuli to the surface membrane, these are effective only at certain points lined up at definite perimeters of each sarcomere (Fig. 36). It seems that stimulation occurs only at those points at which certain branches of the reticular system (the triads) come into contact with the fiber surface. At those points, a brief depolarization of the cell membrane is able to elicit a local contraction that is confined to the protein filaments of one sarcomere and spreads inward toward the center if the surface depolarization is increased in amplitude; there is no sign of a self-regenerating, or all-or-none, response of the contractile apparatus of a sarcomere. This is also evident from the graded relation between membrane potential and active tension developed by muscle fibers when they are exposed to depolarizing, potassium-rich solutions (Hodgkin and Horowicz, 1960).

To summarize, in muscle fibers, the specific response, namely, development of mechanical force and movement, is initiated by a rapid depolarization of the cell membrane in the form of a propagated action potential or a widely distributed neuromuscular junction potential. This electric membrane change becomes effective

figure 36

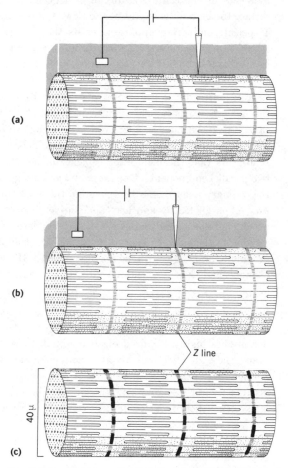

(a)

(b)

Z line

40 μ

(c)

Local activation of contraction by focal depolarization of fiber surface in frog muscle. Shortening is elicited only at certain points along the Z lines indicated by black dots in (c).

through a series of intermediate steps about which we have as yet only fragmentary knowledge. In large skeletal muscle fibers, a special system of intracellular membranous tubes is provided, probably for the purpose of conducting excitation inward and so reducing the distance between the points of electrical change and those of chemical and mechanical response. Reactions involving calcium ions and, subsequently, the splitting of ATP, ultimately lead to an interaction between myosin and actin filaments and so to the development of muscular force.

It is interesting to note certain features that the initiation of muscle contraction shares with the initiation of an action potential and with the release of a transmitter substance at a nerve terminal. In all three cases, the primary event is a depolarization of the cell membrane. Depolarization, however, is not a sufficient stimulus; it becomes effective in producing its diverse results only if calcium is present, whether the final result be increase of sodium permeability (Hodgkin, 1958), the facilitated release of acetylcholine quanta (Katz, 1962), or the activation of myosin molecules (A. F. Huxley, 1964).

12
conclusion

In this brief textbook a number of problems of cellular excitation have been discussed—some in detail and others more superficially. For an introductory treatment, it was thought best to focus attention on the few points that have been clarified by existing experimental evidence, to mention briefly residual uncertainties, and to avoid dealing at length with problems whose solution remains so uncertain that even the most detailed discussion could do no more than assign dubious marks to rival hypotheses.

It is difficult to forecast the direction in which the most fruitful research in neuromuscular and synaptic physiology will be. The major advances and deficiencies in our present knowledge are fairly obvious. Many of the classical descriptive terms, such as "threshold," "action potential," "refractory period," "accommodation," "inhibition," and "excitation," are to a large extent understood in terms of the physical chemistry of cell membranes, and they could, if one wished, be replaced by more scientific (though less convenient) language.

On the other hand, we are still dealing with unknown entities (e.g., "receptors," "ion pumps," "carriers") when we speak of the chemical reactions that are the basis of excitation and synaptic transmission. Furthermore, our preoccupation with rapid electrical methods, which are so eminently suited to the study of impulses and short-term synaptic events, has not enabled us to find a way of approach to the great problems of long-term interactions and modifications in the nervous system. The microchemistry of nervous function is still in its infancy, though some powerful methods are beginning to be developed (Hydén, 1960; Hydén and Egyhazi, 1962; Hydén and Hamberger, 1963). In the meantime, the traditional microelectrical methods will no doubt yield many interesting results and disclose unexpected connections between neuronal pathways and reveal new synaptic mechanisms. It is to be hoped, however, that advances in microchemistry will "catch up" and make an increasing contribution to the study of the nervous system.

references

ADRIAN, E. D. (1928): "The basis of sensation: the action of the sense organs," 122 pp., Christophers Ltd., London.

—— (1932): "The mechanism of nervous action," 103 pp., Oxford University Press, London.

—— (1947): "The physical background of perception," 95 pp., Clarendon Press, Oxford.

ADRIAN, R. H. (1956): The effect of internal and external potassium concentration on the membrane potential of frog muscle, *J. Physiol. (London)*, vol. 133, pp. 631–658.

AUGER, D., and A. FESSARD (1935): Sur une variation négative graduable et non propagée obtenue par stimulation sous-liminaire d'une cellule végétale, *Compt. Rend. Soc. Biol.*, vol. 118, pp. 1059–1060.

AXELSSON, J., and S. THESLEFF (1959): A study of supersensitivity in denervated mammalian skeletal muscle, *J. Physiol. (London)*, vol. 147, pp. 178–199.

BAKER, P. F., A. L. HODGKIN, and T. I. SHAW (1962): Replacement of the axoplasm of giant nerve fibres with artificial solutions, *J. Physiol. (London)*, vol. 164, pp. 330–354.

BENNETT, M. V. L., E. ALJURE, Y. NAKAJIMA, and G. D. PAPPAS (1963): Electrotonic junctions between teleost spinal neurons: electrophysiology and ultrastructure, *Science*, vol. 141, pp. 262–264.

BERNSTEIN, J. (1902): Untersuchungen zur Thermodynamik der bioelektrischen Ströme, *Pflügers Arch. Ges. Physiol.*, vol. 92, pp. 521–562.

BIRKS, R., B. KATZ, and R. MILEDI (1960): Physiological and structural changes at the amphibian myoneural junction, in the course of nerve degeneration, *J. Physiol. (London)*, vol. 150, pp. 145–168.

BIRKS, R. I., and F. C. MACINTOSH (1957): Acetylcholine metabolism at nerve-endings, *Brit. Med. Bull.*, vol. 13, pp. 157–161.

——, and —— (1961): Acetylcholine metabolism of a sympathetic ganglion, *Can. J. Biochem.*, vol. 39, pp. 787–827.

BOISTEL, J., and P. FATT (1958): Membrane permeability change during transmitter action in crustacean muscle, *J. Physiol. (London)*, vol. 144, pp. 176–191.

BOYD, I. A., and A. R. MARTIN (1956): The end-plate potential in mammalian muscle, *J. Physiol. (London)*, vol. 132, pp. 74–91.

BOYLE, P. J., and E. J. CONWAY (1941): Potassium accumulation in muscle and associated changes, *J. Physiol. (London)*, vol. 100, pp. 1–63.

BROCK, L. G., J. S. COOMBS, and J. C. ECCLES (1952): The recording of potentials from motoneurones with an intracellular electrode, *J. Physiol. (London)*, vol. 117, pp. 431–469.

BROOKS, V. B. (1956): An intracellular study of the action of repetitive nerve volleys and of botulinum toxin on miniature end-plate potentials, *J. Physiol. (London)*, vol. 134, pp. 264–277.

BROWN, G. L., H. H. DALE, and W. FELDBERG (1936): Reactions of the normal mammalian muscle to acetylcholine and eserine, *J. Physiol. (London)*, vol. 87, pp. 394–424.

BULLOCK, T. H. (1959): Initiation of nerve impulses in receptor and central neurons, in "Biophysical Sciences–A Study Program," pp. 504–514, John Wiley & Sons, Inc., New York.

BURKE, W., and B. L. GINSBORG (1956): The action of the neuromuscular transmitter on the slow fibre membrane, *J. Physiol. (London)*, vol. 132, pp. 599–610.

BURNSTOCK, G., and M. E. HOLMAN (1961): The transmission of excitation from autonomic nerve to smooth muscle, *J. Physiol. (London)*, vol. 155, pp. 115–133.

———, and ——— (1962): Effect of denervation and of reserpine treatment on transmission at sympathetic nerve endings, *J. Physiol. (London)*, vol. 160, pp. 461–469.

CALDWELL, P. C., A. L. HODGKIN, R. D. KEYNES, and T. I. SHAW (1960): The effects of injecting "energy-rich" phosphate compounds on the active transport of ions in the giant axons of *Loligo*, *J. Physiol. (London)*, vol. 152, pp. 561–590.

COLE, K. S. (1940): Permeability and impermeability of cell membranes for ions, *Cold Spring Harbor Symp. Quant. Biol.*, vol. 8, pp. 110–122.

——— (1949): Dynamic electrical characteristics of the squid axon membrane, *Arch. Sci. Physiol.*, vol. 3, pp. 253–258.

COLE, K. S., and H. J. CURTIS (1939): Electric impedance of the squid giant axon during activity, *J. Gen. Physiol.*, vol. 22, pp. 649–670.

COLE, K. S., and A. L. HODGKIN (1939): Membrane and protoplasm resistance in the squid giant axon, *J. Gen. Physiol.*, vol. 22, pp. 671–687.

CONNELLY, C. M. (1959): Recovery processes and metabolism of nerve, in "Biophysical Sciences–A Study Program," pp. 475–484, John Wiley & Sons, Inc., New York.

CONWAY, B. E. (1952): "Electrochemical data," 374 pp., Elsevier Publishing Company, Amsterdam.

CONWAY, E. J. (1950): Calculation of the idiomolar value and its electrostatic equivalent in normal mammalian skeletal muscle, *Irish J. Med. Sci.*, ser. 6, no. 293, pp. 216–224.

——— (1957): Nature and significance of concentration relations of potassium and sodium ions in skeletal muscle, *Physiol. Rev.*, vol. 37, pp. 84–132.

CONWAY, E. J., R. P. KERNAN, and J. A. ZADUNAISKY (1961): The sodium pump in skeletal muscle in relation to energy barriers, *J. Physiol. (London)*, vol. 155, pp. 263–279.

COOMBS, J. S., J. C. ECCLES, and P. FATT (1955): The specific ionic conductances and the ionic movements across the motoneuronal membrane that produce the inhibitory post-synaptic potential, *J. Physiol. (London)*, vol. 130, pp. 326–373.

COUTEAUX, R. (1955): Localization of cholinesterases at neuromuscular junctions, *Intern. Rev. Cytol.*, vol. 4, pp. 335–375.

CURTIS, H. J., and K. S. COLE (1942): Membrane resting and action potentials from the squid giant axon, *J. Cellular Comp. Physiol.*, vol. 19, pp. 135–144.

DALE, H. H., W. FELDBERG, and M. VOGT (1936): Release of acetylcholine at voluntary motor nerve endings, *J. Physiol. (London)*, vol. 86, pp. 353–380.

DAVSON, H., and J. F. DANIELLI (1943): "The permeability of natural membranes," 361 pp., Cambridge University Press, London.

DEE, E., and R. P. KERNAN (1963): Energetics of sodium transport in *Rana pipiens*, *J. Physiol. (London)*, vol. 165, pp. 550–558.

DEL CASTILLO, J., and L. ENGBAEK (1954): The nature of the neuromuscular block produced by magnesium, *J. Physiol. (London)*, vol. 124, pp. 370–384.

DEL CASTILLO, J., and B. KATZ (1954a): Quantal components of the end-plate potential, *J. Physiol. (London)*, vol. 124, pp. 560–573.

———, and ——— (1954b): Changes in end-plate activity produced by pre-synaptic polarization, *J. Physiol. (London)*, vol. 124, pp. 586–604.

———, and ——— (1954c): The membrane change produced by the neuromuscular transmitter, *J. Physiol. (London)*, vol. 125, pp. 546–565.

———, and ——— (1955a): On the localization of acetylcholine receptors, *J. Physiol. (London)*, vol. 128, pp. 157–181.

———, and ——— (1955b): Local activity at a depolarized nerve-muscle junction, *J. Physiol. (London)*, vol. 128, pp. 396–411.

———, and ——— (1956a): Biophysical aspects of neuromuscular transmission, *Progr. Biophys. Biophys. Chem.*, vol. 6, pp. 121–170.

———, and ——— (1956b): Localization of active spots within the neuromuscular junction of the frog, *J. Physiol. (London)*, vol. 132, pp. 630–649.

———, and ——— (1957a): A study of curare action with an electrical micromethod, *Proc. Roy. Soc. (London)*, ser. B, vol. 146, pp. 339–356.

———, and ——— (1957b): Interaction at end-plate receptors between different choline derivatives, *Proc. Roy. Soc. (London)*, ser. B, vol. 146, pp. 369–381.

DEL CASTILLO, J., and L. STARK (1952): Local responses in single medullated nerve fibres, *J. Physiol. (London)*, vol. 118, pp. 207–215.

DE LORENZO, A. J. (1959): The fine structure of synapses, *Biol. Bull.* 117, p. 390.

DE ROBERTIS, E. (1962): Fine structure of synapses in the CNS, *Intern. Congr. Neuropathol.*, vol. 2, pp. 35–38.

——— (1964): Electron microscope and chemical study of binding sites of brain biogenic amines, *Progr. Brain Res.*, vol. 8, pp. 118–136.

DE ROBERTIS, E., A. PELLEGRINO DE IRALDI, G. RODRIGUEZ, and C. J. GOMEZ (1961): On the isolation of nerve endings and synaptic vesicles, *J. Biophys. Biochem. Cytol.*, vol. 9, pp. 229–235.

DESMEDT, J. E. (1953): Electrical activity and intracellular sodium concentration in frog muscle, *J. Physiol. (London)*, vol. 121, pp. 191–205.

DUDEL, J. (1962): Effect of inhibition on the presynaptic nerve terminal in the neuromuscular junction of the crayfish, *Nature (London)*, vol. 193, pp. 587–588.

DUDEL, J., and S. W. KUFFLER (1961a): The quantal nature of transmission and spontaneous miniature potentials at the crayfish neuromuscular junction, *J. Physiol. (London)*, vol. 155, pp. 514–529.

———, and ——— (1961b): Mechanism of facilitation at the crayfish neuromuscular junction, *J. Physiol. (London)*, vol. 155, pp. 530–542.

———, and ——— (1961c): Presynaptic inhibition at the crayfish neuromuscular junction, *J. Physiol. (London)*, vol. 155, pp. 543–562.

DUDEL, J., and R. K. ORKAND (1960): Spontaneous potential changes at crayfish neuromuscular junctions, *Nature (London)*, vol. 186, pp. 476–477.

DUNHAM, E. T., and I. M. GLYNN (1961): Adenosine triphosphatase activity and the active movements of alkali metal ions, *J. Physiol. (London)*, vol. 156, pp. 274–293.

EBASHI, S., and F. LIPMANN (1962): Adenosine triphosphate-linked concentration of calcium ions in a particulate fraction of rabbit muscle, *J. Cell Biol.*, vol. 14, pp. 389–400.

ECCLES, J. C. (1957): "The physiology of nerve cells," 270 pp., The Johns Hopkins Press, Baltimore.

——— (1961a): The Ferrier Lecture. The nature of central inhibition, *Proc. Roy. Soc. (London)*, Ser. B., vol. 153, pp. 445–476.

——— (1961b): The mechanism of synaptic transmission, *Ergeb. Physiol. Biol. Chem. Exp. Pharmakol.*, vol. 51, pp. 299–430.

——— (1964): "The physiology of synapses," 316 pp., Springer-verlag OHG, Berlin.

ECCLES, J. C., P. FATT, and K. KOKETSU (1954): Cholinergic and inhibitory synapses in a pathway from motor-axon collaterals to motoneurones, *J. Physiol. (London)*, vol. 126, pp. 524–562.

ECCLES, J. C., B. KATZ, and S. W. KUFFLER (1941): Nature of the "endplate potential" in curarized muscle, *J. Neurophysiol.*, vol. 4, pp. 362–387.

ELLIOTT, T. R. (1904): On the action of adrenalin, *J. Physiol. (London)*, vol. 31, p. 20 P.

ELMQVIST, D., D. M. J. QUASTEL, and S. THESLEFF (1963): Prejunctional action of HC-3 on neuromuscular transmission, *J. Physiol. (London)*, vol. 167, pp. 47–48 P.

EMMELIN, N. G., and F. C. MACINTOSH (1956): The release of acetylcholine from perfused sympathetic ganglia and skeletal muscles, *J. Physiol. (London)*, vol. 131, pp. 477–496.

ERNST, E. (1958): "Die Muskeltätigkeit. Versuch einer Biophysik des quergestreiften Muskels," 355 pp., Hungarian Academy of Science, Budapest.

EULER, U. S. VON (1946): A specific sympathomimetic ergone in adrenergic nerve fibres (Sympathin) and its relations to adrenaline and noradrenaline, *Acta Physiol. Scand.*, vol. 12, pp. 73–97.

EYZAGUIRRE, C., and S. W. KUFFLER (1955): Processes of excitation in the dendrites and in the soma of single isolated nerve cells of the lobster and crayfish, *J. Gen. Physiol.*, vol. 39, pp. 87–119.

FALK, G., and P. FATT (1964): Linear electrical properties of striated muscle fibres observed with intracellular electrodes, *Proc. Roy. Soc. (London)*, ser. B, vol. 160, pp. 69–123.

FATT, P. (1957a): Electric potentials occurring around a neuron during its antidromic activation, *J. Neurophysiol.*, vol. 20, pp. 27–60.

——— (1957b): Sequence of events in synaptic activation of a motoneuron, *J. Neurophysiol.*, vol. 20, pp. 61–80.

FATT, P., and B. L. GINSBORG (1958): The ionic requirements for the production of action potentials in crustacean muscle fibres, *J. Physiol.*, *(London)*, vol. 142, pp. 516–543.

FATT, P., and B. KATZ (1950): Some observations on biological noise, *Nature (London)*, vol. 166, pp. 597–598.

———, and ——— (1951): An analysis of the end-plate potential recorded with an intracellular electrode, *J. Physiol. (London)*, vol. 115, pp. 320–370.

———, and ——— (1952): Spontaneous subthreshold activity at motor nerve endings, *J. Physiol. (London)*, vol. 117, pp. 109–128.

———, and ——— (1953): The effect of inhibitory nerve impulses on a crustacean muscle fibre, *J. Physiol. (London)*, vol. 121, pp. 374–389.

FENG, T. P., and W. M. HSIEH (1952a): Conduction in muscle after complete irreversible inactivation of cholinesterase, *Chinese J. Physiol.*, vol. 18, pp. 81–92.

———, and ——— (1952b): Conduction in nerve after complete irreversible inactivation of cholinesterase, *Chinese J. Physiol.*, vol. 18, pp. 93–102.

FENG, T. P., and T. H. LI (1941): Studies on the neuromuscular junction, XXIII, A new aspect of the phenomena of eserine potentiation and post-tetanic facilitation in mammalian muscles, *Chinese J. Physiol.*, vol. 16, pp. 37–56.

FRANK, K (1959): Basic mechanisms of synaptic transmission in the central nervous system, *IRE Trans. Med. Electron.*, vol. ME-6, pp. 85–88.

FRANK, K., and M. G. F. FUORTES (1957): Presynaptic and postsynaptic inhibition of monosynaptic reflexes, *Federation Proc.*, vol. 16, pp. 39–40.

FRANKENHAEUSER, B. (1952): The hypothesis of saltatory conduction, *Cold Spring Harbor Symp. Quant. Biol.*, vol. 17, pp. 27–36.

——— (1960): Quantitative description of sodium currents in myelinated nerve fibres of *Xenopus laevis*, *J. Physiol. (London)*, vol. 151, pp. 491–501.

FRANKENHAEUSER, B., and A. L. HODGKIN (1956): The after-effects of impulses in the giant nerve fibres of *Loligo*, *J. Physiol. (London)*, vol. 131, pp. 341–376.

FRANZINI-ARMSTRONG, C., and K. R. PORTER (1964): Sarcolemmal invaginations constituting the T system in fish muscle fibres, *J. Cell Biol.*, vol. 22, pp. 675–696.

FUORTES, M. G. F., K. FRANK, and M. C. BECKER (1957): Steps in the production of motoneuron spikes, *J. Gen. Physiol.*, vol. 40, pp. 735–752.

FURSHPAN, E. J., and T. FURUKAWA (1962): Intracellular and extracellular responses of the several regions of the Mauthner cell of the goldfish, *J. Neurophysiol.*, vol. 25, pp. 732–771.

FURSHPAN, E. J., and D. D. POTTER (1959): Transmission at the giant synapses of the crayfish, *J. Physiol. (London)*, vol. 145, pp. 289–325.

FURUKAWA, T., and E. J. FURSHPAN (1963): Two inhibitory mechanisms in the Mauthner neurons of goldfish, *J. Neurophysiol.*, vol. 26, pp. 140–176.

GAFFEY, C. T., and L. J. MULLINS (1958): Ion fluxes during the action potential in *Chara*, *J. Physiol.* (*London*), vol. 144, pp. 505–524.

GEREN, B. B. (1954): The formation from the Schwann cell surface of myelin in the peripheral nerves of chick embryos, *Exper. Cell Res.*, vol. 7, pp. 558–562.

GLYNN, I. M. (1962): Activation of adenosine-triphosphatase activity in a cell membrane by external potassium and internal sodium, *J. Physiol.* (*London*), vol. 160, pp. 18–19 P.

GOLDMAN, D. E. (1943): Potential, impedance and rectification in membranes, *J. Gen. Physiol.*, vol. 27, pp. 37–60.

GOLDSMITH, T. H. (1963): Rates of action of bath-applied drugs at the neuromuscular junction of the frog, *J. Physiol.* (*London*), vol. 165, pp. 368–386.

GRANIT, R. (1955): "Receptors and sensory perception," 369 pp., Yale University Press, New Haven, Conn.

GRAY, E. G., and V. P. WHITTAKER (1962): The isolation of nerve endings from brain: an electron microscope study of cell fragments derived by homogenization and ultracentrifugation, *J. Anat.* (*London*), vol. 96, pp. 79–88.

GRAY, J. A. B. (1959): Initiation of impulses at receptors, chap. 4 of "Neurophysiology," vol. 1, Section 1, "Handbook of Physiology," J. Field (ed.), pp. 123–145, American Physiol Society, Washington, D. C., 1959.

GRUNDFEST, H. (1957): Electrical inexcitability of synapses and some consequences in the central nervous system, *Physiol. Rev.*, vol. 37, pp. 337–361.

HAGIWARA, S., and I. TASAKI (1958): A study of the mechanism of impulse transmission across the giant synapse of the squid, *J. Physiol.* (*London*), vol. 143, pp. 114–137.

HAMA, K. (1961): Some observations on the fine structure of the giant fibres of the crayfishes (*Cambarus virilis* and *Cambarus clarkii*) with special reference to the sub-microscopic organization of the synapses, *Anat. Record*, vol. 141, pp. 275–280.

——— (1962): Some observations on the fine structure of the giant synapse in the stellate ganglion of the squid, *Doryteuphis bleekeri*, *Z. Zellforsch.*, vol. 56, pp. 437–444.

HANSON, J., and H. E. HUXLEY (1955): The structural basis of contraction in striated muscle, *Symp. Soc. Exptl. Biol.*, vol. 9, pp. 228–264.

———, and ——— (1957): Quantitative studies on the structure of cross-striated myofibrils, II, Investigations by biochemical analysis, *Biochem. Biophys. Acta.*, vol. 23, pp. 250–260.

HARRIS, E. J., and G. P. BURN (1949): The transfer of sodium and potassium ions between muscle and the surrounding medium, *Trans. Faraday Soc.*, vol. 45, pp. 508–528.

HARTLINE, H. K. (1959): Receptor mechanisms and the integration of sensory information in the eye, in "Biophysical Science—A Study Program," pp. 515–523, John Wiley & Sons, Inc., New York.

HASSELBACH, W., and M. MAKINOSE (1961): Die Calciumpumpe der "Er-schlaffungsgrana" des Muskels und ihre Abhängigkeit von der ATP-Spaltung, *Biochem. Z.*, vol. 333, pp. 518–528.

HILL, A. V. (1932): "Chemical wave transmission in nerve," 74 pp., Cambridge University Press, London.

—— (1938): The heat of shortening and the dynamic constants of muscle, *Proc. Roy. Soc. (London)*, ser. B, vol. 126, pp. 136–195.

—— (1949): The onset of contraction, *Proc. Roy. Soc. (London)*, ser. B, vol. 136, pp. 242–254.

—— (1956): The thermodynamics of muscle, *Brit. Med. Bull.*, vol. 12, pp. 174–176.

HINKE, J. A. M. (1961): The measurement of sodium and potassium activities in the squid axon by means of cation-selective glass micro-electrodes, *J. Physiol. (London)*, vol. 156, pp. 314–335.

HODGKIN, A. L. (1937): Evidence for electrical transmission in nerve, *J. Physiol. (London)*, vol. 90, pp. 183–232.

—— (1938): The subthreshold potentials in a crustacean nerve fibre, *Proc. Roy. Soc. (London)*, ser. B, vol. 126, pp. 87–121.

—— (1951): The ionic basis of electrical activity in nerve and muscle, *Biol. Rev.*, vol. 26, pp. 339–409.

—— (1954): A note on conduction velocity, *J. Physiol. (London)*, vol. 125, pp. 221–224.

—— (1958): The Croonian Lecture: Ionic movements and electrical activity in giant nerve fibres, *Proc. Roy. Soc. (London)*, ser. B, vol. 148, pp. 1–37.

—— (1964): "The conduction of the nervous impulse," 108 pp., Liverpool University Press, Liverpool.

HODGKIN, A. L., and P. HOROWICZ (1959): Movements of Na and K in single muscle fibres, *J. Physiol. (London)*, vol. 145, pp. 405–432.

——, and —— (1960): Potassium contractures in single muscle fibres, *J. Physiol. (London)*, vol. 153, pp. 386–403.

HODGKIN, A. L., and A. F. HUXLEY (1939): Action potentials recorded from inside a nerve fibre, *Nature (London)*, vol. 144, p. 710.

——, and —— (1952a): Movement of sodium and potassium ions during nervous activity, *Cold Spring Harbor Symp. Quant. Biol.*, vol. 17, pp. 43–52.

——, and —— (1952b): Currents carried by sodium and potassium ions through the membrane of the giant axon of *Loligo*, *J. Physiol. (London)*, vol. 116, pp. 449–472.

——, and —— (1952c): The components of membrane conductance in the giant axon of *Loligo*, *J. Physiol. (London)*, vol. 116, pp. 473–496.

——, and —— (1952d): The dual effect of membrane potential on sodium conductance in the giant axon of *Loligo*, *J. Physiol. (London)*, vol. 116, pp. 497–506.

——, and —— (1952e): A quantitative description of membrane current and its application to conduction and excitation in nerve, *J. Physiol. (London)*, vol. 117, pp. 500–544.

HODGKIN, A. L., A. F. HUXLEY, and B. KATZ (1949): Ionic currents underlying activity in the giant axon of the squid, *Arch. Sci. Physiol.*, vol. 3, pp. 129–150.

——, ——, and —— (1952): Measurement of current-voltage relations in the membrane of the giant axon of *Loligo*, *J. Physiol. (London)*, vol. 116, pp. 424–448.

HODGKIN, A. L., and B. KATZ (1949): The effect of sodium ions on the electrical activity of the giant axon of the squid, *J. Physiol. (London)*, vol. 108, pp. 37–77.

HODGKIN, A. L., and R. D. KEYNES (1953): The mobility and diffusion coefficient of potassium in giant axons from *Sepia*, *J. Physiol. (London)*, vol. 119, pp. 513–528.

——, and —— (1955a): Active transport of cations in giant axons from *Sepia* and *Loligo*, *J. Physiol. (London)*, vol. 128, pp. 28–60.

——, and —— (1955b): The potassium permeability of a giant nerve fibre, *J. Physiol. (London)*, vol. 128, pp. 61–88.

HODGKIN, A. L., and W. A. H. RUSHTON (1946): The electrical constants of a crustacean nerve fibre, *Proc. Roy. Soc. (London)*, ser. B, vol. 133, pp. 444–479.

HOYLE, G., and C. A. G. WIERSMA (1958): Inhibition at neuromuscular junctions in crustacea, *J. Physiol. (London)*, vol. 143, pp. 426–440.

HUXLEY, A. F. (1957): Muscle structure and theories of contraction, *Progr. Biophys. Biophys. Chem.*, vol. 7, pp. 255–318.

—— (1964): Muscle, *Ann. Rev. Physiol.*, vol. 26, pp. 131–152.

HUXLEY, A. F., and R. STÄMPFLI (1949): Evidence for saltatory conduction in peripheral myelinated nerve fibres, *J. Physiol. (London)*, vol. 108, pp. 315–339.

——, and —— (1951): Effect of potassium and sodium on resting and action potentials of single myelinated nerve fibres, *J. Physiol. (London)*, vol. 112, pp. 496–508.

HUXLEY, A. F., and R. E. TAYLOR (1958): Local activation of striated muscle fibres, *J. Physiol. (London)*, vol. 144, pp. 426–441.

HUXLEY, H. E. (1957): The double array of filaments in cross-striated muscle, *J. Biophys. Biochem. Cytol.*, vol. 3, pp. 631–648.

—— (1960): "Muscle cells," in "The Cell," vol. 4, pp. 366–481, Academic Press, Inc., New York.

—— (1963): Electron microscope studies on the structure of natural and synthetic protein filaments from striated muscle, *J. Mol. Biol.*, vol. 7, pp. 281–308.

HYDÉN, H. (1960): "The neuron," in "The Cell," vol. 4, pp. 215–323, Academic Press, Inc., New York.

HYDÉN, H., and E. EGYHAZI (1962): Nuclear RNA changes of nerve cells during a learning experiment in rats, *Proc. Natl. Acad. Sci. U.S.*, vol. 48, pp. 1366–1373.

HYDÉN, H., and A. HAMBERGER (1963): Inverse enzymatic changes in neurons and glia during increased function and hypoxia, *J. Cell Biol.*, vol. 16, pp. 521–525.

JENKINSON, D. H. (1960): The antagonism between tubocurarine and substances which depolarize the motor end-plate, *J. Physiol. (London)*, vol. 152, pp. 309–324.

KATCHALSKY, A. (1954): Polyelectrolyte gels, *Progr. Biophys. Biophys. Chem.*, vol. 4, pp. 1–59.

KATZ, B. (1937): Experimental evidence for a non-conducted response of nerve to subthreshold stimulation, *Proc. Roy. Soc. (London)*, ser. B, vol. 124, pp. 244–276.

———— (1939): "Electric excitation of nerve," 151 pp., Oxford University Press, London.

———— (1947): Subthreshold potentials in medullated nerve, *J. Physiol. (London)*, vol. 106, pp. 66–79.

———— (1948): The electrical properties of the muscle fibre membrane, *Proc. Roy. Soc. (London)*, ser. B, vol. 135, pp. 506–534.

———— (1950): Depolarization of sensory terminals and the initiation of impulses in the muscle spindle, *J. Physiol. (London)*, vol. 111, pp. 261–283.

———— (1958): Microphysiology of the neuromuscular junction, *Johns Hopkins Hosp. Bull.*, vol. 102, pp. 275–312.

———— (1960): Book review, *Perspectives Biol. Med.*, vol. 3, pp. 563–565.

———— (1961): The terminations of the afferent nerve fibre in the muscle spindle of the frog, *Phil. Trans. Roy. Soc. London*, ser. B, vol. 243, pp. 221–240.

———— (1962): The Croonian Lecture: The transmission of impulses from nerve to muscle, and the subcellular unit of synaptic action, *Proc. Roy. Soc. (London)*, ser. B, vol. 155, pp. 455–477.

KATZ, B., and R. MILEDI (1963): A study of spontaneous miniature potentials in spinal motoneurones, *J. Physiol. (London)*, vol. 168, pp. 389–422.

————, and ———— (1964a): The development of acetylcholine sensitivity in nerve-free segments of skeletal muscle, *J. Physiol. (London)*, vol. 170, pp. 389–396.

————, and ———— (1964b): Localization of calcium action at the nerve muscle junction, *J. Physiol. (London)*, vol. 171, pp. 10–12 *P*.

————, and ———— (1965a): Propagation of electric activity in motor nerve terminals, *Proc. Roy. Soc. (London)*, ser. B, vol. 161, pp. 453–482.

————, and ———— (1965b): The measurement of synaptic delay, and the time course of acetylcholine release at the neuromuscular junction, *Proc. Roy. Soc. (London)*, ser. B, vol. 161, pp. 483–495.

————, and ———— (1965c): The effect of calcium on acetylcholine release from motor nerve terminals, *Proc. Roy. Soc. (London)*, ser. B, vol. 161, pp. 496–503.

KATZ, B., and O. H. SCHMITT (1940): Electric interaction between two adjacent nerve fibres, *J. Physiol. (London)*, vol. 97, pp. 471–488.

KATZ, B., and S. THESLEFF (1957a): On the factors which determine the amplitude of the "miniature end-plate potential," *J. Physiol. (London)*, vol. 137, pp. 267–278.

————, and ———— (1957b): The interaction between edrophonium (tensilon) and acetylcholine at the motor end-plate, *Brit. J. Pharmacol.*, vol. 12, pp. 260–264.

————, and ———— (1957c): A study of the "desensitization" produced by acetylcholine at the motor end-plate, *J. Physiol. (London)*, vol. 138, pp. 63–80.

KERKUT, G. A., and R. C. THOMAS (1964): The effect of anion injection and changes in the external potassium and chloride concentration on the reversal potentials of the IPSP and acetylcholine, *Comp. Biochem. Physiol.*, vol. 11, pp. 199–213.

KEYNES, R. D. (1951): The ionic movements during nervous activity, *J. Physiol. (London)*, vol. 114, pp. 119–150.

—— (1954): The ionic fluxes in frog muscle, *Proc. Roy. Soc. (London)*, ser. B, vol. 142, pp. 359–382.

KEYNES, R. D., and P. R. LEWIS (1951): The sodium and potassium content of cephalopod nerve fibres, *J. Physiol. (London)*, vol. 114, pp. 151–182.

KEYNES, R. D., and G. W. MAISEL (1954): The energy requirement for sodium extrusion from a frog muscle, *Proc. Roy. Soc. (London)*, ser. B, vol. 142, pp. 383–392.

KOELLE, G. B., and J. S. FRIEDENWALD (1949): A histochemical method for localizing cholinesterase activity, *Proc. Soc. Exptl. Biol. Med.*, vol. 70, pp. 617–622.

KRAVITZ, E. A., S. W. KUFFLER, and D. D. POTTER (1963): Gamma-aminobutyric acid and other blocking compounds in Crustacea, III, Their relative concentrations in separated motor and inhibitory axons, *J. Neurophysiol.*, vol. 26, pp. 739–751.

KRNJEVIĆ, K., and R. MILEDI (1958): Failure of neuromuscular propagation in rats, *J. Physiol. (London)*, vol. 140, pp. 440–461.

KRNJEVIĆ, K., and J. F. MITCHELL (1961): The release of acetylcholine in the isolated rat diaphragm, *J. Physiol. (London)*, vol. 155, pp. 246–262.

KUFFLER, S. W. (1942): Further study on transmission in an isolated nerve-muscle fibre preparation, *J. Neurophysiol.*, vol. 5, pp. 309–322.

—— (1949): Transmitter mechanism at the nerve-muscle junction, *Arch. Sci. Physiol.*, vol. 3, pp. 585–601.

—— (1960): Excitation and inhibition in single nerve cells, "The Harvey Lectures, 1958–1959," pp. 176–218, Academic Press Inc., New York.

KUFFLER, S. W., and D. D. POTTER (1964): Glia in the leech central nervous system: physiological properties and neuron-glia relationship, *J. Neurophysiol.*, vol. 27, pp. 290–320.

KUFFLER, S. W., and E. M. VAUGHAN WILLIAMS (1953): Small-nerve junctional potentials: The distribution of small motor nerves to frog skeletal muscle, and the membrane characteristics of the fibres they innervate, *J. Physiol. (London)*, vol., 121, pp. 289–317.

KUNO, M. (1964): Quantal components of excitatory synaptic potentials in spinal motoneurones, *J. Physiol. (London)*, vol. 175, pp. 81–99.

LEVI, H., and H. H. USSING (1948): The exchange of sodium and chloride ions across the fibre membrane of the isolated frog sartorius, *Acta Physiol. Scand.*, vol. 16, pp. 232–249.

LILEY, A. W. (1956a): The quantal components of the mammalian endplate potential, *J. Physiol. (London)*, vol. 133, pp. 571–587.

—— (1956b): The effects of presynaptic polarization on the spontaneous activity of the mammalian neuromuscular junction, *J. Physiol. (London)*, vol. 134, pp. 427–443.

LILLIE, R. S. (1936): The passive iron wire model of protoplasmic and nervous transmission and its physiological analogies, *Biol. Rev.*, vol. 11, pp. 181–209.

LING, G. N. (1962): "A physical theory of the living state," 680 pp., Blaisdell Publishing Company, New York.

LOEWI, O. (1921): Über humorale Übertragbarkeit der Herznervenwirkung, *Pflügers Arch. Ges. Physiol.*, vol. 189, pp. 239–242.

LOEWI, O., and E. NAVRATIL (1926): Über humorale Übertragbarkeit der Herznervenwirkung, X., Über das Schicksal des Vagusstoffes, *Pflügers Arch. Ges. Physiol.*, vol. 214, pp. 678–688.

LORENTE DE NÓ, R. (1947): "A study of nerve physiology," *Studies Rockefeller Inst. Med. Res.*, vol. 131, 496 pp., and vol. 132, 548 pp.

LORENTE DE NÓ, R., and G. A. CONDOURIS (1959): Decremental conduction in peripheral nerve. Integration of stimuli in the neuron, *Proc. Nat. Acad. Sci., U.S.*, vol. 45, pp. 592–617.

LÜTTGAU, H. C., and R. NIEDERGERKE (1958): The antagonism between Ca and Na ions on the frog's heart, *J. Physiol. (London)*, vol. 143, pp. 486–505.

MAKAROV, P., and N. JUDENICH (1929): On the conduction of the nerve impulse in a narcotized nerve segment, *J. Exp. Biol. Med.* (Moscow), vol. 11, pp. 65–69.

MARRAZZI, A. S., and R. LORENTE DE NÓ (1944): Interaction of neighboring fibers in myelinated nerve, *J. Neurophysiol.*, vol. 7, pp. 83–102.

MARTIN, A. R. (1955): A further study of the statistical composition of the end-plate potential, *J. Physiol. (London)*, vol. 130, pp. 114–122.

MARTIN, A. R., and R. K. ORKAND (1961): Postsynaptic effects of HC-3 at the neuromuscular junction of the frog, *Can. J. Biochem. Physiol.*, vol. 39, pp. 343–349.

MARTIN, A. R., and G. PILAR (1963a): Dual mode of synaptic transmission in the avian ciliary ganglion, *J. Physiol. (London)*, vol. 168, pp. 443–463.

———, and ——— (1963b): Transmission through the ciliary ganglion of the chick, *J. Physiol. (London)*, vol. 168, pp. 464–475.

MASLAND, R. L., and R. S. WIGTON (1940): Nerve activity accompanying fasciculation produced by prostigmine, *J. Neurophysiol.*, vol. 3, pp. 269–275.

MATTHEWS, B. H. C. (1931): The response of a single end-organ, *J. Physiol. (London)*, vol. 71, pp. 64–110.

MILEDI, R. (1960a): The acetylcholine sensitivity of frog muscle fibres after complete or partial denervation, *J. Physiol. (London)*, vol. 151, pp. 1–23.

——— (1960b): Properties of regenerating neuromuscular synapses in the frog, *J. Physiol. (London)*, vol. 154, pp. 190–205.

——— (1962): Induction of receptors, in "Enzymes and drug action," pp. 220–238, J. and A. Churchill, Ltd., London.

——— (1963): An influence of nerve not mediated by impulses, in E. Gutmann and P. Hnik (eds.) "The effect of use and disuse on neuromuscular functions," pp. 35–41, Czechoslovak Academy of Sciences, Prague.

MILEDI, R., and C. R. SLATER (1963): A study of rat nerve-muscle junctions after degeneration of the nerve, *J. Physiol. (London)*, vol. 169, pp. 23–24 P.

NACHMANSOHN, D. (1959): "Chemical and molecular basis of nerve activity," 235 pp., Academic Press, Inc., New York.

NASTUK, W. L. (1953): Membrane potential changes at a single muscle endplate produced by transitory application of acetylcholine with an electrically controlled microjet, *Federation Proc.*, vol. 12, p. 102.

NASTUK, W. L., and A. L. HODGKIN (1950): The electrical activity of single muscle fibres, *J. Cellular Comp. Physiol.*, vol. 35, pp. 39–74.

OVERTON, E. (1902): Beiträge zur allgemeinen Muskel- und Nervenphysiologie, II, Über die Unentbehrlichkeit von Natrium- (oder Lithium-) Ionen für den Kontraktionsakt des Muskels. *Pflügers Arch. Ges. Physiol.*, vol. 92, pp. 346–386.

PALAY, S. L. (1956): Synapses in the central nervous system, *J. Biophys. Biochem. Cytol.*, vol. 2, pp. 193–202.

POST, R. L., C. R. MERRITT, C. R. KINSOLVING, and C. D. ALBRIGHT (1960): Membrane adenosine-triphosphatase as a participant in the active transport of sodium and potassium in the human erythrocyte, *J. Biol. Chem.*, vol. 235, pp. 1796–1802.

RANDIĆ, M., and D. W. STRAUGHAN (1964): Antidromic activity in the rat phrenic nerve-diaphragm preparation. *J. Physiol. (London)*, vol. 173, pp. 130–148.

RITCHIE, J. M., and R. W. STRAUB (1957): The hyperpolarization which follows activity in mammalian non-medullated fibres, *J. Physiol. (London)*, vol. 136, pp. 80–97.

ROBERTSON, J. D. (1960): The molecular structure and contact relationship of cell membranes, *Progr. Biophys. Biophys. Chem.*, vol. 10, pp. 343–418.

——— (1961): Ultrastructure of excitable membranes and the crayfish median-giant synapse, *Ann. N.Y. Acad. Sci.*, vol. 94, pp. 339–389.

ROSENBLUETH, A. (1950): "The transmission of nerve impulses at neuroeffector junctions and peripheral synapses," 325 pp., John Wiley & Sons, Inc., New York.

——— (1952): The local responses of axons, *Ergeb. Physiol. Biol. Chem. Exp. Pharmakol.*, vol. 47, pp. 24–69.

RUSHTON, W. A. H. (1932): A new observation in the excitation of nerve and muscle, *J. Physiol. (London)*, vol. 75, pp. 16–17 P.

——— (1951): A theory of the effects of fibre size in medullated nerve, *J. Physiol. (London)*, vol. 115, pp. 101–122.

SCHATZMANN, A. J. (1953): Herzglykoside als Hemmstoffe für den aktiven Kalium und Natriumtransport durch die Erythrocytenmembran, *Helv. Physiol. Acta.*, vol. 11, pp. 346–354.

SCHMITT, F. O. (1959): Molecular organization of the nerve fiber, in "Biophysical Science–A Study Program," pp. 455–465, John Wiley & Sons, Inc., New York.

SCHMITT, O. H. (1959): Biological transducers and coding, in "Biophysical Science–A Study Program," pp. 492–503, John Wiley & Sons, Inc., New York.

SJÖSTRAND, F. S. (1959): Fine structure of cytoplasm: the organization of membranous layers, in "Biophysical Science–A Study Program," pp. 301–318, John Wiley & Sons, Inc., New York.

SKOU, J. C. (1957): The influence of some cations on an adenosinetriphosphatase from peripheral nerves. *Biochim. biophys. acta*, vol. 23, pp. 394–401.

STÄMPFLI, R. (1958): Reversible electrical breakdown of the excitable membrane of the Ranvier node, *Anais Acad. Brasil. Cienc.*, vol. 30, pp. 57–63.

STEINBACH, H. B. (1940): Sodium and potassium in frog muscle, *J. Biol. Chem.*, vol. 133, pp. 695–701.

SZENT-GYÖRGYI, A. (1947): "Chemistry of muscular contraction," 150 pp., Academic Press Inc., New York.

TAKEUCHI, A., and N. TAKEUCHI (1959): Active phase of frog's end-plate potential, *J. Neurophysiol.*, vol. 22, pp. 395–411.

———, and ——— (1960*a*): On the permeability of end-plate membrane during the action of transmitter, *J. Physiol. (London)*, vol. 154, pp. 52–67.

———, and ——— (1960*b*): Further analysis of relationship between end-plate potential and end-plate current, *J. Neurophysiol.*, vol. 23, pp. 397–402.

———, and ——— (1964): The effect on crayfish muscle of iontophoretically applied glutamate, *J. Physiol. (London)*, vol. 170, pp. 296–317.

TASAKI, I. (1939): The electro-saltatory transmission of the nerve impulse and the effect of narcosis upon the nerve fiber, *Am. J. Physiol.*, vol. 127, pp. 211–227.

——— (1953): "Nervous Transmission," p. 164, Charles C Thomas, Publisher, Springfield, Ill.

TAUC, L. (1958): Processus post-synaptique d'excitation et d'inhibition dans le soma neuronique de L'Aplysie et de l'Escargot, *Arch. Ital. Biol.*, vol. 96, pp. 78–110.

TAUC, L., and H. M. GERSCHENFELD (1961): Cholinergic transmission mechanisms for both excitation and inhibition in molluscan central synapses, *Nature (London)*, vol. 192, pp. 366–367.

———, and ——— (1962): A cholinergic mechanism of inhibitory synaptic transmission in a molluscan nervous system, *J. Neurophysiol.*, vol. 25, pp. 236–262.

THESLEFF, S. (1955): The mode of neuromuscular block caused by acetylcholine, nicotine, decamethonium and succinylcholine, *Acta Physiol. Scand.*, vol. 34, pp. 218–231.

——— (1960*a*): Supersensitivity of skeletal muscle produced by botulinum toxin, *J. Physiol. (London)*, vol. 151, pp. 598–607.

——— (1960*b*): Effects of motor innervation on the chemical sensitivity of skeletal muscle, *Physiol. Rev.*, vol. 40, pp. 734–752.

THIES, R. E., and V. B. BROOKS (1961): Postsynaptic neuromuscular block produced by hemicholinium No. 3, *Federation Proc.*, vol. 20, pp. 569–578.

TROSCHIN, A. S. (1958): "Das Problem der Zellpermeabilität," 396pp., Gustav Fischer Verlag, Jena.

——— (1960): Concerning an article by L. M. Chailakhian—Modern concepts of the nature of the resting potential, *Biophysics (USSR)*, Eng. transl., vol. 5, pp. 104–111.

USSING, H. H. (1947): Interpretation of the exchange of radiosodium in isolated muscle, *Nature (London)*, vol. 160, pp. 262–263.

———— (1949): Transport of ions across cellular membranes, *Physiol. Rev.*, vol. 29, pp. 127–155.

WEBER, A., R. HERZ, and I. REISS (1963): On the mechanism of the relaxing effect of fragmented sarcoplasmic reticulum, *J. Gen. Physiol.*, vol. 46, pp. 679–702.

WHITTAKER, V. P. (1964): Investigations on the storage sites of biogenic amines in the central nervous system, *Progr. Brain Res.*, vol. 8, pp. 90–117.

WHITTAM, R. (1958): Potassium movements and ATP in human red cells, *J. Physiol. (London)*, vol. 140, pp. 479–497.

WIERSMA, C. A. G. (1941): The efferent innervation of muscle, *Biol. Symp.*, vol. 3, pp. 259–290.

index

Catalog

If you are interested in a list of fine Paperback
books, covering a wide range of subjects
and interests, send your name and address,
requesting your free catalog, to:

McGraw-Hill Paperbacks
330 West 42nd Street
New York, New York 10036